T0326320

Curbside
Consultation
of the Foot and Ankle

49 Clinical Questions

CURBSIDE CONSULTATION IN ORTHOPEDICS
SERIES

SERIES EDITOR, BERNARD R. BACH, JR, MD

Curbside Consultation
of the Foot and Ankle

49 Clinical Questions

EDITED BY

George B. Holmes, Jr, MD
Assistant Professor
Director
Foot & Ankle Section
Department of Orthopaedic Surgery
Rush University Medical Center
Chicago, Illinois

Simon Lee, MD
Assistant Professor
Department of Orthopaedic Surgery
Rush University Medical Center
Midwest Orthopaedics at Rush
Chicago, Illinois

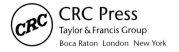

CRC Press
Taylor & Francis Group
Boca Raton   London   New York

CRC Press is an imprint of the
Taylor & Francis Group, an **informa** business

First published 2012 by SLACK Incorporated

Published 2024 by CRC Press
2385 NW Executive Center Drive, Suite 320, Boca Raton FL 33431

and by CRC Press
4 Park Square, Milton Park, Abingdon, Oxon, OX14 4RN

CRC Press is an imprint of Taylor & Francis Group, LLC

Library of Congress Cataloging-in-Publication Data

Curbside consultation of the foot and ankle : 49 clinical questions / edited by George B. Holmes Jr., Simon Lee.
     p. ; cm. -- (Curbside consultation in orthopedics series)
   Includes bibliographical references and index.
    ISBN 9781556429392 (pbk. : alk. paper)
   I. Holmes, George B. II. Lee, Simon, 1971- III. Series: Curbside consultation in orthopedics.
   [DNLM: 1. Foot Diseases--diagnosis. 2. Foot Diseases--therapy. 3. Ankle Injuries--diagnosis. 4. Ankle Injuries--therapy. 5. Foot Deformities--diagnosis. 6. Foot Deformities--therapy. WE 880]

   616.579--dc23

                        2011039867

ISBN: 9781556429392 (pbk)
ISBN: 9781003523741 (ebk)

DOI: 10.1201/9781003523741

Dedication

To my wife, Ann, and my children, Cori and Anisa, for their love, support, and patience.

To my parents, Gloria Holmes and the late George B. Holmes, for their love and inspiration.

To Dr. Roger Mann for his intellectual and scholarly mentorship.

George B. Holmes, Jr, MD

To my parents, who strived to achieve the best they could for their children.

To my children, Lauren, Amanda, and Parker.

Finally, but most importantly, to my wife, Audrey, for her love, patience, and support through my career.

Simon Lee, MD

Contents

Acknowledgments

I would like to convey my deepest gratitude to each of the contributors for their efforts and diligence. Very special thanks go to Dr. Simon Lee for his organizational skills and enthusiastic support of this project. All of the contributors are indebted to the professionalism, persistence, and vision of Dr. Bernard Bach, Dani Karaszkiewicz (Project Editor), April Billick (Managing Editor), Carrie Kotlar (Senior Aquisitions Editor), Nikki Best (Marketing Coordinator), and SLACK Incorporated.

George B. Holmes, Jr, MD

My thanks go to the following:

My partner, Bernie Bach, and SLACK Incorporated for giving me the opportunity to publish *Curbside Consultation of the Foot and Ankle.*

Drs. Edward Abraham, Steve Kodros, and Armen Kelikian for initiating my interest in a career in foot and ankle and literally and figuratively getting my foot in the door.

My mentors in Charlotte for teaching me the highest level of care and the continued education and knowledge throughout my career.

Simon Lee, MD

About the Editors

George B. Holmes, Jr, MD graduated from Yale College in New Haven, Connecticut and earned his medical degree from Yale University School of Medicine. He completed his orthopedic residency at the Harvard Combined Orthopaedic Residency. This was followed by a sports medicine fellowship with Lyle Micheli, MD at the Children's Hospital Boston in Massachusetts and a foot and ankle fellowship with Roger A. Mann, MD in Oakland, California.

Dr. Holmes is currently Director of the Section of Foot & Ankle Surgery at Rush University Medical Center, Chicago, Illinois. He is also an editor for *Foot & Ankle International* and has hosted visiting fellows from Brazil and Poland. Past nonacademic activities include serving as an orthopedic consultant for the Joffrey Ballet, the Philadelphia Dance Company, the Boston Marathon, the Chicago Bulls, and the Sacramento Kings. He has authored numerous peer-reviewed and nonpeer-reviewed articles; regional, national and international podium presentations; and book chapters.

Simon Lee, MD is an assistant professor in Orthopaedic Surgery at Rush University Medical College. He is a graduate of Rush Medical College, completing his orthopedic surgery residency at the University of Illinois, Chicago. He completed his Foot and Ankle Surgery Fellowship in Charlotte, North Carolina at the Miller Clinic and Carolina's Medical Center.

Dr. Lee is active in the continued education of orthopedic residents at Rush Medical Center in foot and ankle surgery. He is active and serves as a committee member for the American Orthopedic Foot and Ankle Society (AOFAS). Dr. Lee has served on the faculty of numerous courses on surgery of the foot and ankle through the AAOS and AOFAS. Additionally, he is a reviewer for the *Foot and Ankle International* (FAI) journal. Locally, Dr. Lee serves as the foot and ankle consultant for numerous Chicago metro area high schools, colleges, semi-professional and professional dance companies, and the Chicago White Sox and Chicago Bulls.

Contributing Authors

Jeremy A. Alland, BA (Questions 29, 30)
Medical Student
Rush Medical College of Rush University
Rush University Medical Center
Chicago, Illinois

John G. Anderson, MD (Questions 11, 13)
Associate Professor
Deptartment of Orthopaedic Surgery
Michigan State University
College of Human Medicine
Assistant Program Director, GRMEP
    Orthopaedic Residency
Co-Director, Grand Rapids Orthopaedic
    Foot and Ankle Fellowship Program
Orthopedic Associates of Michigan
Grand Rapids, Michigan

Robert B. Anderson, MD (Questions 27, 33)
Chief, Foot and Ankle
Carolinas Medical Center
OrthoCarolina
Charlotte, North Carolina

Judith Baumhauer, MD, MPH (Questions 7, 34)
Associate Chair of Academic Affairs
Professor, Department of Orthopaedics
University of Rochester School of Medicine
    and Dentistry Department
Rochester, New York

Wayne Berberian, MD (Questions 10, 14)
Vice Chair
Associate Professor
Department of Orthopaedics
New Jersey Medical School
Newark, New Jersey

Gregory C. Berlet, MD (Questions 17, 24)
Orthopedic Foot and Ankle Center
Westerville, Ohio

Christopher Bibbo, DO, FACS, FAAOS (Questions 16, 49)
Chief, Foot & Ankle Section
Department of Orthopaedics
Marshfield Clinic
Clinical Instructor, Department of Surgery
University of Wisconsin School of Medicine
    & Public Health
Marshfield, Wisconsin

Donald R. Bohay, MD, FACS (Questions 5, 19)
Associate Clinical Professor
Department of Orthopaedic Surgery
Michigan State University
College of Human Medicine
Lansing, Michigan
Private Practice
Orthopedic Associates of Michigan
Grand Rapids, Michigan

Eric Breitbart, MD (Questions 10, 14)
Orthopaedic Resident
Department of Orthopaedics
New Jersey Medical School
Newark, New Jersey

Yong Chae, DPM, FACFAS (Question 6)
Private Practice
Indianapolis, Indiana

Christopher P. Chiodo, MD (Questions 31, 44)
Chief, Foot and Ankle Division
Brigham and Women's Hospital
Harvard Medical School
Boston, Massachusetts

Jennifer Chu, MD (Questions 7, 34)
Orthopaedic Resident
Department of Orthopaedic Surgery
University of Rochester School of Medicine
    and Dentistry
Rochester, New York

Cara A. Cipriano, MD (Question 42)
Resident Physician
Department of Orthopaedics
Rush University Medical Center
Chicago, Illinois

Bruce Cohen, MD (Questions 9, 28)
Fellowship Director
OrthoCarolina Foot and Ankle Institute
Charlotte, North Carolina

W. Hodges Davis, MD (Questions 20, 26)
Medical Director
OL Foot and Ankle Institute at Mercy
OrthoCarolina
Charlotte, North Carolina

Nickolas G. Garbis, MD (Question 35)
PGY-5 Resident in Orthopedics
Rush University Medical Center
Department of Orthopedic Surgery
Chicago, Illinois

Jaymes D. Granata, MD (Questions 17, 24, 37, 43)
Resident
Department of Orthopaedics
The Ohio State University Medical Center
Columbus, Ohio

Robert R. L. Gray, MD (Question 25)
Assistant Professor
Division of Hand and Microvascular Surgery
Department of Orthopaedic Surgery
Miller School of Medicine
University of Miami
Miami, Florida

Carroll P. Jones, MD (Questions 36, 47)
OrthoCarolina Foot and Ankle Fellowship
Carolinas Medical Center
Charlotte, North Carolina

Armen S. Kelikian, MD (Questions 12, 23)
Professor of Orthopedics
Northwestern University Medical School
Department of Orthopedics
Chicago, Illinois

Alex J. Kline, MD (Question 27)
Orthopedic Foot and Ankle Fellow
Three Rivers Orthopedic Associates-UPMC
Pittsburgh, Pennsylvania

Pradeep Kodali, MD (Questions 22, 39)
Orthopaedic Sports Medicine
Assistant Professor
Department of Orthopaedic Surgery
University of Texas Health Sciences Center at Houston
Ironman Sports Medicine Institute
Houston, Texas

Steven A. Kodros, MD (Questions 4, 18)
Associate Professor of Clinical Orthopaedic Surgery
Department of Orthopaedic Surgery
Northwestern University Feinberg School of Medicine
Chicago, Illinois

Johnny Lin, MD (Questions 35, 45)
Orthopaedic Foot and Ankle Specialist
Midwest Orthopaedics at Rush
Chicago, Illinois

Sheldon Lin, MD (Questions 10, 14)
Associate Professor
Department of Orthopaedics
New Jersey Medical School
Newark, New Jersey

Sameer J. Lodha, MD (Question 41)
Resident
Department of Orthopaedic Surgery
Rush University Medical Center
Chicago, Illinois

Robert S. Marsh, DO (Questions 5, 19)
OrthoIndy
Indianapolis, Indiana

Samuel McArthur, MD (Questions 40, 45)
Orthopedic Resident
Rush University Medical Center
Chicago, IL

Scott Nemec, DO (Questions 11, 13)
Bay Street Orthopaedics
Petoskey Michigan
Clinical Assistant Professor
Department of Osteopathic Surgical
  Specialties
Michigan State University
College of Osteopathic Medicine
East Lansing, Michigan

Shane J. Nho, MD, MS (Questions 29, 30)
Assistant Professor of Orthopedic Surgery
Rush Medical College of Rush University
Department of Orthopedic Surgery
Rush University Medical Center
Chicago, Illinois

Daniel L. Ocel, MD (Questions 1, 3)
Cornerstone Orthopedics and Sports
  Medicine
Foot and Ankle Service
Louisville, Colorado

Terrence M. Philbin, DO (Questions 37, 43)
Director
Foot and Ankle Service
Doctors Hospital Residency
Columbus, Ohio
Attending Physician
Orthopedic Foot and Ankle Center
Westerville, Ohio

Michael S. Pinzur, MD (Questions 8, 46)
Professor of Orthopaedic Surgery
Loyola University Health System
Maywood, Illinois

David R. Richardson, MD (Questions 2, 15)
Program Director
Department of Orthopaedic Surgery
University of Tennessee-Campbell Clinic
Memphis, Tennessee

Nicholas R. Seibert, MD (Question 33)
Private Practice
Orthopedic Physician Associates
Seattle, Washington

Brian C. Toolan, MD (Questions 32, 38)
Professor of Surgery
Section of Orthopaedic Surgery and
  Rehabilitation Medicine
The University of Chicago Pritzker School
  of Medicine
Director, Foot & Ankle Service
University of Chicago Medical Center
Chicago, Illinois

Walter W. Virkus, MD (Questions 41, 42)
Associate Professor
Residency Program Director
Department of Orthopedic Surgery
Rush University Medical Center
Chicago, Illinois

Anand Vora, MD (Questions 22, 39)
Orthopaedic Foot and Ankle Surgery
Illinois Bone & Joint Institute
Assistant Clinical Professor of Orthopedics
University of Illinois Medical School
Chicago, Illinois

Keith L. Wapner, MD (Questions 21, 48)
Clinical Professor of Orthopedic Surgery
University of Pennsylvania
Adjunct Professor of Orthopedic Surgery
Drexel University College of Medicine
Philadelphia, Pennsylvania

Preface

Curbside Consultation of the Foot and Ankle reflects the rapid growth of the orthopedic interest and understanding of the complexities of the foot and ankle. The American Orthopaedic Foot and Ankle Society has been one of the fastest growing societies within the orthopedic community.

Curbside Consultation of the Foot and Ankle provides a means of forming a bridge between the growing body of research and clinical data related to the foot and ankle and the real world challenges that confront the clinicians providing foot and ankle care in the community.

George B. Holmes, Jr, MD
Midwest Orthopaedics at Rush
Chicago, IL

Foreword

Experience is the mother of knowledge. –Nicholas Breton

So much can be learned from the experiences of others, and this collaboration of 49 "situational" chapters epitomizes that. Drs. Holmes and Lee have worked diligently to create realistic patient scenarios that provide an interesting framework for foot and ankle experts to teach.

Who says that reading for education has to be boring? The chapters included in this text are quite the opposite, using a more anecdotal type of writing style that provides the reader a more relaxed manner in which to relate to the disorder at hand. It's a fun way to learn.

The reader will find that the most common of foot and ankle problems are addressed within the text, equally distributed from forefoot to ankle, but each with its own little curveball. Symptomatic sesamoid stress fractures, recurrent Morton's neuroma, and a subacute Achilles tendon rupture are problems that do not present to even the busy foot and ankle subspecialist on a regular basis. However, the chapters are written with appropriate background information so that the scenerios are applicable to the daily setting.

The topics are nicely arranged in sections, which include an excellent list of timely sport- and trauma-related issues. The authors selected by the editors are diverse in background; they are products of a wide variety of fellowship "camps" and also represent both academic and private practice interests.

It is a true pleasure and honor to have been associated with this text. This is a "must" for those physicians managing a wide variety of foot and ankle problems, and regardless of their years of experience or exposure to this subspecialty. I believe that this will be a valuable reference for those surgeons practicing in some degree of isolation and without the benefit of colleagues to exchange ideas. The chapters will alleviate fears and hesitations one may have if unfamiliar with a certain topic. It truly does serve as a "curbside" consultation without having to pick up the phone or fire off an email.

I commend Drs. Holmes and Lee on a very successful educational product—one that is uniquely creative in thought and yet quite practical in content. As we all know, there are a number of different approaches to solving a problem and this book should help the surgeon find the most direct route.

Robert B. Anderson, MD
Chief, Foot and Ankle
Carolinas Medical Center
OrthoCarolina
Charlotte, North Carolina

—

SECTION I

FOREFOOT/MIDFOOT

HOW DO YOU EVALUATE AND TREAT AN 18-YEAR-OLD FEMALE WITH PLANTAR HALLUX METATARSOPHALANGEAL PAIN AND A RADIOLUCENT LINE ON HER SESAMOID?

Daniel L. Ocel, MD

When evaluating the patient with a complaint of plantar first metatarsophalangeal (MTP) joint pain, a thorough history and physical examination is warranted. Often, a single precipitating event is not reported and therefore an evaluation of sports participation, training habits, as well as dietary habits, particularly in the female, is imperative. Participation in running activities or dance, particularly ballet activities, may focus the clinician on possible underlying etiology of the pain and, in particular, to a sesamoid injury.

The importance of the metatarsal sesamoid complex in the appropriate function of the hallux cannot be overemphasized. Anatomically, the sesamoids are contained within the tendons of the flexor hallucis brevis (FHB) and serve to elevate the metatarsal head, thereby increasing the mechanical advantage of the FHB and other forefoot intrinsics. The sesamoids also absorb and dissipate forces placed upon the first ray. In addition, they serve to protect the flexor hallucis longus tendon, which runs directly between the sesamoids, thereby maintaining its direct pull upon the phalanx.

Evaluating the individual's gait pattern as well as visualizing the alignment of the lower extremity and foot begins the physical examination. Evaluating the patient for subtle versus overt cavus is quite important. Assess alignment and mobility of the first ray because a plantarflexed first ray can lead to overload of the metatarsal sesamoid complex. This can be assessed with physical examination as well as more specified use of the Coleman block test. Performing a Silfverskiöld test assessing for gastroc equinus is likewise important in the investigation of underlying causes. Typical physical findings include diminished range of motion of the first MTP joint and pain to direct palpation of the sesamoids individually. Plantar medial pain is more typical for tibial sesamoid involvement and direct lateral plantar pain is more typical of fibular sesamoid involvement.

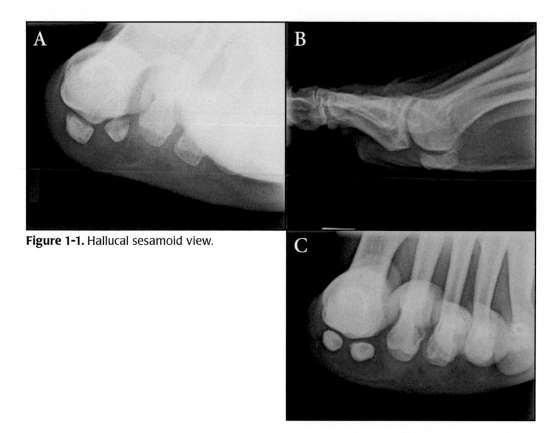

Figure 1-1. Hallucal sesamoid view.

Radiographic evaluation should be undertaken and include weight-bearing anteroposterior, lateral, and oblique views. The oblique view is particularly useful in evaluating the tibial sesamoid. The axial or sesamoid view is likewise valuable (Figure 1-1). I have also found that placement of a radiographic BB marker placed over the point of maximum tenderness is particularly useful in helping differentiate particular sesamoid involvement or other nonsesamoid pathology.

Bipartite sesamoids should always be considered when one notes radiolucency on the radiograph, particularly of the tibial sesamoid. Multiple studies have shown the incidence of bipartite tibial sesamoids to be anywhere from 10% to 35%. The tibial sesamoid is involved nearly 10 times more commonly versus its fibular counterpart. Bilaterality of the bipartite sesamoid is likewise quite common, and one study by Zinman and colleagues noted a 90% incidence of bilaterality.[1]

Advanced imaging studies are very useful, particularly regarding a bipartite sesamoid and whether it is symptomatic. Studies have shown that congenitally bipartite sesamoids fracture with much less force then nonbipartite sesamoids. Bone scans, although having a higher rate of false positives, can demonstrate increased uptake prior to developing significant plain radiographic changes. I typically do not obtain an MRI on the initial evaluation but will consider this imaging modality if the pain is recalcitrant. I find MRI useful to differentiate soft tissue from bony pathology as well as sesamoid viability.

My initial treatment protocol depending on the severity of the injury or pain is nonoperative. For milder injuries, an initial period of immobilization with a boot or a cast for 7 to 10 days followed by compression taping to limit motion and anti-inflammatories followed by orthotic evaluation and shoe modifications are appropriate. I have the patient assessed for a custom foot orthotic using a carbon fiber Morton's extension. In addition, maintaining a low heel height will help diminish pressure across the first MTP joint.

For acute fractures, I opt for casting and nonweight bearing until the fracture is healed, typically 6 to 8 weeks. I modify the cast with a toe spica extension, placing the MTP joint in mild plantarflexion.

When conservative management fails to provide satisfactory relief of the first MTP pain over a period of 3 to 4 months, surgical options may be entertained and include autogenous bone grafting and repair or excision. Anderson and McBryde described autogenous bone grafting of the tibial sesamoid in which they bone grafted nonunions with positive bone scans who failed conservative management for 6 months.[2] They noted that the procedure was technically demanding and unfortunately had variable results.

Surgical consideration likewise includes complete surgical excision of the offending sesamoid that remains unresponsive to conservative management. Should complete excision be considered, one must be aware of concomitant foot deformities such as hallux valgus, claw toe, stiffness within the MTP joint, as well as possible cavus hindfoot deformity.

My preference is to use an extra-articular approach to the tibial sesamoid if possible. I make a longitudinal incision that is placed slightly plantar to that for a standard hallux valgus correction. Localization of the plantar medial digital nerve is essential. A longitudinal capsular incision just above the abductor hallucis tendon is performed, exposing the MTP joint. Assessment of both the MTP joint as well as the articular surface of the sesamoid should be performed and at this point, one can make the decision to proceed with bone grafting or a sesamoidectomy. I then repair the capsule and proceed with an extra-articular excision performed through the same incision, which will allow repair of the FHB after removal. A Beaver blade (#69; BD Medical, Franklin Lakes, NJ) is quite helpful in subperiosteal excision of the sesamoid circumferentially. A subsequent side-to-side repair or "purse string" repair with absorbable suture is then performed on the defect.

For the fibular sesamoid, I use a plantar curvilinear incision off the weight-bearing pad of the MTP. Once again, it is imperative to identify the plantar lateral nerve. Shelling out of the fibular sesamoid with a Beaver blade and possible release of the adductor tendon with repair of the FHB is performed.

My postoperative protocol for tibial sesamoid excision is heel weight bearing until the 2 week point and, after suture removal, a bunion spacer and weight bearing as tolerated in either a postoperative shoe or short walker boot until the 8-week postoperative point. Due to the plantar-based incision, I maintain the fibular sesamoid excision on nonweight-bearing status until suture removal at the 3-week point. The protocol is similar to that for a tibial sesamoidectomy.

References

1. Zinman H, Keret D, Reis N. Fracture of the medial sesamoid bone of the hallux. *J Trauma*. 1981;21(7):581-582.
2. Anderson RB, McBryde AM Jr. Autogenous bone grafting of hallux sesamoid nonunions. *Foot Ankle Int*. 1997;18:293-296.

MY MOTHER-IN-LAW IS DEVELOPING PROGRESSIVE PAIN IN THE BALL OF HER FOOT AND CLAWING OF HER LESSER TOES. WHAT DO I DO?

David R. Richardson, MD

Forefoot pain is a common complaint in patients seen by foot and ankle specialists.[1-6] While metatarsalgia in general can be frustrating to both the patient and physician, the differential can usually be narrowed to a couple of possibilities. At that point, the success or failure of conservative treatment will help tease out a final diagnosis. It is important to have a good working differential in patients with metatarsalgia (Table 2-1).

As with most entities, a thorough history is vital to understanding the underlying pathology. First, have the patient remove both shoes and socks before hearing his or her history. This will allow you to begin to observe both the symptomatic and, hopefully, asymptomatic side. Try to get a feel for the onset of symptoms. Did the pain begin acutely or gradually? What about the onset of the deformity? Next, ask about the nature of the pain. Is it sharp, achy, burning? Does it worsen with weight bearing? Does the style of shoe or wearing shoes at all affect the pain? Is the pain affected by how the patient stands or sits? Ask about other joint complaints that may lead you to a diagnosis of systemic arthritis or other disease (eg, multiple sclerosis).

Next, move on to the physical exam. Perform a good neurovascular exam. You would not be the first physician to miss pain or deformity of the foot associated with spinal stenosis or other lumbar pathology. Be sure your mother-in-law does not have claudication or neuropathy. Examine her heel cord because a tight Achilles tendon is associated with increased forefoot pressure. Note whether she has pain on her metatarsal (MT) neck or in the web space. Only then, press directly on the metatarsophalangeal (MTP) joint of the affected digit. This will probably produce the greatest amount of discomfort and will make the rest of the exam more difficult if not already completed.[2,6] I have found that plantarflexion of the MTP joint also helps with the diagnosis, reproduction of pain, and recreation of the patient's symptoms. An interdigital neuroma produces minimal pain, while the opposite occurs with MTP synovitis. The drawer sign (sagittal manipulation

---

Table 2-1

Differential Diagnosis of Metatarsalgia

Synovitis	Radiculopathy
Inflammatory arthritis	Infection
MT stress fracture	Freiberg's infraction
Web space neuroma	Sesamoiditis
Keratotic lesion	MT fat pad atrophy
Plantar wart	Trauma (fracture/dislocation)
Neuropathy	Autoimmune diseases

---

of the MTP joint) will also elicit characteristic pain and can help quantitate the amount of instability at the MTP joint. Note if there is a callus under the MT head.[2,3] If so, is it painful to palpation? While a callus may indicate pressure overload, if it is not painful to palpation, the relevant pathology is probably elsewhere. It is important to differentiate at which joint the deformity is occurring—the distal interphalangeal (DIP), proximal inter-phalangeal (PIP), or MTP joint.[5,6] Also test for the flexibility of the deformity to determine if it is passively reducible. If there is a bunion, decide if this may have contributed to the lesser toe deformity.

Standing radiographs of the foot are the only imaging required at the initial visit. Three views of the foot will demonstrate the extent of joint subluxation or dislocation as well as any hallux deformity. Changes in the MT head, such as those associated with Freiberg's infraction, can also be noted. A long second digit relative to the first as well as hallux valgus deformity may increase pressure on the second MTP joint, causing synovitis, capsular stretching, and eventually pain and deformity.[1-6]

Your mother-in-law is describing a deformity associated with pain in the fat pad of her forefoot. She most likely has ruptured her plantar plate leading to extension of the MTP joint, thus placing the intrinsic muscles (primarily the lumbricals) at a biomechanical disadvantage, leading to more significant extension deformity and a claw toe. The pain is associated with excess pressure under her MT head. She also likely has pain directly in her MTP joint associated with synovitis or irritation of the joint capsule. In patients with bunions, the second digit is often the most symptomatic.

Because the pain and presumably the deformity are progressive, the deformity will probably be flexible.[2,5,6] If this is the case, begin treatment by showing her how to plan-tarflex tape her MTP joint (Figure 2-1). If the bunion interferes with reduction, you can use a toe spacer in the first web space to help. Any conversation concerning forefoot pain requires you to have a serious discussion with the patient (your mother-in-law) about shoe wear. A wide toe-box and soft uppers are necessary, at least in the short term. She will also need pressure relief under her painful MT head, which may be accomplished by offload-ing the pressure area with an MT support (Figure 2-2A) or padding the MT head (Figure 2-2B). I have found that off-the-shelf inserts are usually effective in relieving pain. I usu-ally add a flexible carbon insert (Figure 2-2C) to stiffen the shoe and prevent a dorsiflexion moment at the forefoot, thus relieving stress on the damaged plantar plate. If there are no

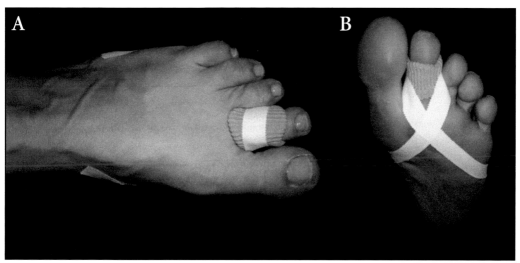

Figure 2-1. Plantarflex taping for metatarsalgia.

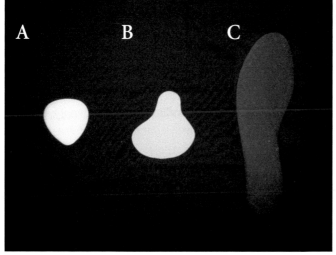

Figure 2-2. (A) MT support. (B) MT pad. (C) Flexible carbon insert.

contraindications, adding a nonsteroidal medication is often beneficial. Alternatively, you can try a tapered dose of steroid such as methylprednisolone (ie, Medrol Dosepak). Symptoms usually improve significantly after 6 weeks of treatment. If she continues to have pain, it is reasonable to try adding a controlled ankle motion walker or even a short leg walking cast with a toe plate. I strongly discourage injecting the joint with steroid. While this will provide you and your mother-in-law almost instant gratification, it will further weaken the damaged plantar structures and joint capsule, leading to a progression of deformity and ultimate worsening of the symptoms.[2,6]

If conservative treatment fails, your mother-in-law may require surgery. Lesser toe surgery often has less-than-perfect results. Rarely does the toe look, feel, and move as it did before injury. Your mother-in-law should have a standard preoperative workup (eg, ensuring appropriate vascularity, general medical health) done. She will need to

<table>
<tr><td colspan="3" align="center">Table 2-2

Procedures for Lesser Toe Deformities</td></tr>
</table>

Deformity	*Characteristics*	*Treatment*
Flexible hammer toe	No fixed contracture at MTP or PIP joint	Usually nonoperative; rarely, flexor-to-extensor transfer using FDL
Rigid hammer toe with MTP subluxation	Fixed flexion contracture at PIP; MTP subluxation in extension	Resection of condyles of proximal phalanx, dermodesis; lengthening of EDL, tenotomy of EDB; MTP capsulotomy, collateral ligament sectioning
Rigid hammer toe with MTP subluxation; claw toe	Fixed flexion contracture at PIP; MTP subluxation in extension	Resection of condyles of proximal phalanx, dermodesis; lengthening of EDL, tenotomy of EDB; MTP capsulotomy, collateral ligament sectioning
Rigid hammer toe with MTP dislocation	Fixed flexion contracture at PIP; complete MTP dislocation	Resection of condyles of proximal phalanx, dermodesis; lengthening of EDL, tenotomy of EDB; MTP capsulotomy, collateral ligament sectioning; MTP arthroplasty or MT shortening osteotomy
Crossover toe	Fixed flexion contracture at PIP; MTP subluxation in varus or valgus	Resection of condyle of proximal phalanx, dermodesis; collateral ligament/capsular repair; EDB transfer; MT shortening osteotomy
Mallet toe	Fixed flexion contracture at DIP	Resection of condyles of middle phalanx, dermodesis; FDL tenotomy

DIP, distal interphalangeal joint; EDB, extensor digitorum brevis; EDL, extensor digitorum longus; FDL, flexor digitorum longus; MT, metatarsal; MTP, metatarsophalangeal joint; PIP, proximal interphalangeal joint.

Adapted from Ishikawa SN, Murphy GA. Lesser toe abnormalities. In: Canale ST, Beaty JH, eds. *Campbell's Operative Orthopaedics.* 11th ed. Philadelphia, PA: Elsevier; 2008:4632.

understand that other procedures not directly related to her lesser toes may be needed. A tight heel cord may need to be released, usually with a gastrocnemius recession, or perhaps a bunion deformity will need to be corrected, even if asymptomatic, to allow room for the second digit to be reduced. She also needs to understand that ischemia may result with any surgery done on the lesser toes, even with good vasculature.

Many procedures are used to correct lesser toe deformity and relieve excessive MT head pressure (Table 2-2). If the deformity is mild, I would plan to release the MTP joint by performing an extensor digitorum brevis (EDB) tenotomy, lengthening the extensor digitorum longus, and releasing the MTP capsule. If this does not correct the extension deformity, you can do a direct repair of the plantar plate (which often is difficult and may require a fairly extensive planter approach). Other options include a flexor-to-extensor transfer (Girdlestone-Taylor procedure) or EDB tendon transfer. A plantar condylectomy will often help relieve the plantar pressure but may result in a transfer of pain to the adjacent MT heads.

If the deformity is more rigid, the MTP joint will need to be decompressed. This can be accomplished by resecting 3 to 4 mm of MT head in addition to a plantar condylectomy (DuVries arthroplasty). The extensor hood can then be interposed in the MTP joint (Myerson's modification) if desired. Another option is an MT shortening osteotomy. A distal oblique osteotomy is made and the MT translated proximally about 4 mm and held with a Kirschner wire or screw.

Postoperatively, your mother-in-law will be in a forefoot dressing and can bear weight as tolerated in a postoperative shoe. Be sure she understands that her foot will be swollen for up to 8 weeks.

References

1. Coughlin MJ. Common causes of pain in the forefoot in adults. *J Bone Joint Surg Br*. 2000;82:781-790.
2. Dockery GL. Evaluation and treatment of metatarsalgia and keratotic disorders. In: Myerson M, ed. *Foot and Ankle Disorders*. Philadelphia, PA: Saunders; 2000:359-377.
3. Espinosa N, Maceira E, Myerson MS. Current concepts review: metatarsalgia. *Foot Ankle Int*. 2008;29:871-879.
4. Fortin PT, Myerson MS. Second metatarsal joint instability. *Foot Ankle Int*. 1995;16:306-313.
5. Ishikawa SN, Murphy GA. Lesser toe abnormalities. In: Canale ST, Beaty JH, eds. *Campbell's Operative Orthopaedics*. 11th ed. Philadelphia, PA: Elsevier; 2008:4632.
6. Scranton PE Jr. Metatarsalgia: diagnosis and treatment. *J Bone Joint Surg Am*. 1980;62:723-732.

MY PATIENT HAS FAILED CONSERVATIVE TREATMENT OF A MORTON'S NEUROMA. DO I PERFORM A PLANTAR OR DORSAL SURGICAL APPROACH?

Daniel L. Ocel, MD

Patients presenting with pain in the forefoot require a thorough assessment as numerous conditions can cause symptoms that require consideration. When considering the diagnosis of an interdigital neuroma, the typical patient complaint is of burning, aching, or shooting pain within the region of the second, third, or fourth metatarsophalangeal (MTP) joints that typically extends plantarward from its dorsal location or proximally within the midfoot. Rarely does the pain extend past the region of the ankle. Most often, the pain is ill defined but at times can be specifically isolated to a central web space. Patients can often state that the pain is related to their shoe wear, relieved by removing of the shoe and massaging of the foot. The most common sources of forefoot pain, which can often be misdiagnosed as an interdigital neuroma are lesser MTP synovitis or metatarsalgia and less common pathologies such as lumbar radiculopathy, peripheral neuropathy, and Freiberg's infraction. The more common entities, however, are typically improved with appropriate shoe wear modifications and exacerbated by barefoot ambulation. Clearly, appropriate and accurate physical examination is essential in the diagnosis of forefoot pain prior to initiating conservative or surgical measures as disappointment after surgical intervention is often the result of a failure to recognize the correct source of the forefoot pain during the initial evaluation.

Typically, the physical examination is initially performed with the patient in a seated position where the toes are examined for splaying, although this may exist with other disorders such as MTP synovitis. This exam includes MTP range of motion, tenderness within the web space using palpation in a proximal to distal fashion in the interspaces, and an evaluation for a positive Mulder's click. Though not always found, Mulder's click strongly supports the suspected diagnosis of an interdigital neuroma, particularly if this recreates the patient's symptomatology. In addition, evaluation of standing and ambulatory mechanics are also performed as correction of possible dynamic abnormalities may indeed prove successful with proper orthotic management. The evaluation should also include standing, anteroposterior, lateral, as well as oblique radiographs to exclude any notable bony pathology for the underlying etiology of the pain. More advanced imaging modalities may be indicated if there is a suspicion for other entities (particularly other neurologic causes for the pain); however, they are rarely necessary in the evaluation of interdigital neuromas.

From my perspective, once the clinical diagnosis of an interdigital neuroma is suspected, a local injection can be quite useful in support of the diagnosis as well as initially providing relief. The patient should be informed about the purpose of the injection mainly from a diagnostic perspective. As noted by Rasmussen and colleagues, most patients obtain relief from the symptoms. However, in 40% of the study population, the symptoms returned and surgical excision was recommended.[1] In my practice, a diagnostic injection is absolutely integral in the initial evaluation and diagnosis of a neuroma, as failure to obtain relief from an interdigital injection should guide the practitioner to evaluate for other entities.

The surgical management of an interdigital neuroma has traditionally involved either excision or decompression neurolysis. Many surgeons prefer surgical excision as the initial surgical treatment of recalcitrant interdigital neuromas. Decompression may be less successful if intrinsic damage is noted to the nerve itself or the neuroma is particularly large, which may result in continued irritation of the nerve.

An interdigital neuroma may be excised through either a plantar or dorsal approach. The main advantage of approaching the neuroma dorsally is avoidance of a painful or hypertrophic scar along the plantar surface of the foot. In a prospective randomized study of 52 patients undergoing an interdigital neuroma excision, those who had undergone a dorsal incision had a higher likelihood of good to excellent results, faster return to weight bearing, as well as a lower incidence of painful scars and faster return to work versus their counterparts who had undergone a plantar incision.[2]

The surgery is typically performed with the patient in a supine position. An ankle block anesthesia is supplemented by light sedation. A sterile supramalleolar Esmarch tourniquet is used. A dorsal incision is started within the web space between the affected toes and is extended proximally 2 to 3 cm. This generally ends up proximal to the metatarsal (MT) heads. The incision is kept between the longitudinal axes of the MTs not in line with the extensor tendons. Typically, I perform the surgery under loupe magnification in order to appropriately perform the dissection and excision. The dissection is deepened through the subcutaneous tissues and the dorsal sensory nerve branches of the superficial peroneal nerve should be identified and retracted gently to the side of least resistance as avoidance of injury to these nerves dorsally may prevent a painful neuroma within the scar. Once the dorsal interosseous fascia is identified in the proximal aspect of the incision, this can be followed distally to the web space and an inflamed interdigital bursa overlying the intermetatarsal ligament can be identified. I find at this point direct plantar pressure on the foot will deliver the neuroma into the dorsal wound assisting in visualizing the nerve. Once the bursa is excised, the intermetatarsal ligament is usually easily identified. The ligament is often more plantarward than one would assume. I typically use a Freer elevator to sweep back proximally along the medial border of the lateral MT, and a laminar spreader is placed between the MT necks such that the ligament is placed on tension when spread. This also facilitates visualization within the deep dissection. I will then use a Senn retractor within the web space, which provides retraction of the distal web space adipose tissue. The intermetatarsal ligament, having been identified distally, is released in a distal-to-proximal fashion. Once again, I typically place a Freer elevator on the plantar surface of the intermetatarsal ligament and release this under direct visualization with a #15 blade. In order to assure complete release, I use digital palpation to confirm release of the entire intermetatarsal ligament. Other aspects of the dissection include the identification of the lumbrical tendon, which typically passes medially to the adjacent proximal phalanx, and the interdigital artery, which usually courses from proximal medial to distal lateral over the nerve itself. Having isolated the nerve, I will then dissect it in a distal-to-proximal circumferential manner. Typically, the muscle belly of the adductor hallucis muscle is encountered and, at times, a small incision in the muscle belly is performed in order to trace the nerve proximally. A Freer or Joker elevator is used to identify the proximal extent of my transection in order to be assured that the area is within the nonweight-bearing portion of the foot and proximal transection is then performed sharply. The nerve will then be traced distally and removed from the web space distal to the bifurcation. It is important not to remove a significant portion of the proximal web space fat as this may also contribute to an unsightly and sensitive scar. I typically send the specimen for pathologic confirmation.

The tourniquet is deflated and I will hold compression for 3 to 5 minutes before re-evaluating for hemostasis. I will apply a bulky, compressive dressing, and the patient is instructed on very strict elevation for the following 2 to 3 days. This is mainly for pain management. Patients are then allowed to weight bear on the heel after this point. Removal of the sutures is performed at 10 to 14 days. The patient has been instructed on care of the incision, particularly with cross frictional massage, and I instruct my patients that they may have some tenderness within the web space for upwards of 2 to 3 months. The patient is maintained in a postoperative shoe for 3 to 4 weeks, and unrestricted use of the foot can be commenced at the 2-month postoperative period.

References

1. Rasmussen MR, Kitaoka HB, Patzer G. Nonoperative treatment of plantar interdigital neuroma with a single corticosteroid injection. *Clin Orthop Relat Res*. 1996;326:188-193.
2. Nashi M, Venkatachalam AK, Muddu BN. Surgery of Morton's neuroma: dorsal or plantar approach? *J R Coll Surg Edinb*. 1997;42:36-37.

A 43-Year-Old Recreational Marathon Runner Is Having Pain Over Her Bunion. Will This Eventually Need Surgery?

Steven A. Kodros, MD

The management of the female recreational marathon runner with a bunion is not too dissimilar from that of bunions on other types of patients. Conservative treatment options are often effective and should be tried before considering surgical intervention. Primary conservative treatment involves attention to the use of accommodative shoe wear. In the case of the patient who has bunion pain related to running, one must evaluate certain aspects of her running shoes. Shoes that are fabricated with decorative seams or stitching located directly over the bunion and producing increased pressure or pain should be avoided. Although most running shoes are fairly well made, there are idiosyncrasies that exist with different models of shoes and manufacturers. Given this, the patient may need to try different shoes in order to find the manufacturer and style of shoe that is most comfortable for her. Orthotic insoles can occasionally be used, particularly if the patient suffers from excessive pronation. One mistake made by patients in an effort to alleviate their symptoms is to lace their running shoes more loosely. This can lead to increased movement or forward sliding of the foot within the shoe, which can in turn aggravate their symptoms or create other problems. One method of alleviating pain that is aggravated by the lacing of the shoe is to initiate the lacing 1 or 2 sets of eyelets back from the distal most pair (Figure 4-1).

Another important consideration to be made in treating the patient with a bunion is to evaluate the patient for other underlying sources of pain. Sesamoid pathology, first metatarsophalangeal joint osteoarthritis or hallux rigidus, and transfer metatarsalgia can occur coexistent with or independent of a bunion and be sources of forefoot pain. A careful physical exam, plain x-rays, and, if necessary, additional imaging studies can help to rule out other causes of forefoot pain.

If the patient presents with functionally limiting pain that is unresponsive to these conservative treatment efforts, surgical intervention is indicated. Algorithms for the

Figure 4-1. Modified shoe lacing.

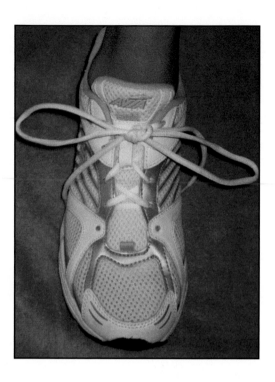

specific surgical treatment of bunions have been described and are generally useful. Although the specific surgical procedure chosen should address the specific character-istics and the severity of the deformity, one should generally try to avoid more extensive forefoot reconstructions in individuals that participate in high-level athletic activity such as distance running. Furthermore, the patient should understand that his or her ability to return to distance running may be limited even after a successful uncomplicated surgical procedure to correct the bunion.

In a patient such as this, if possible, I prefer to surgically correct the bunion with a distal first metatarsal chevron osteotomy. This procedure offers advantages of a relatively rapid recovery, a good rate of healing and correction of deformity, a low rate of transfer metatarsalgia and other complications, generally less stiffness, and a fairly high-level patient satisfaction. This procedure can be performed under regional ankle block anes-thesia. A midline medial incision overlying the first metatarsal phalangeal joint and metatarsal head is used to avoid injury to the dorsal cutaneous nerve. The medial capsule is exposed and an inverted L-shaped capsulotomy is performed. The medial capsule and subperiosteal tissues are elevated off of the medial eminence. An oscillating saw is used to perform a minimal resection of the medial eminence in line with the medial border of the foot. Care should be taken to stay medial to the medial sesamoid sulcus with this resection. A lateral soft tissue release can be performed either transarticular or through a separate dorsal first web space incision if indicated. The oscillating saw is then used to create an apex distal V-shaped chevron osteotomy in the metatarsal head. The distal (capital) segment of the metatarsal is then translated laterally approximately 4 mm and the osteotomy reduced with axial compression. Internal fixation of the osteotomy is generally indicated and can be accomplished with either a Kirschner wire, bioabsorb-able pin, or screw depending on surgeon preference. Remaining excess medial bone is

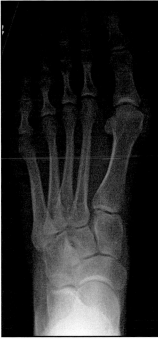

Figure 4-2. Bunion and hallux valgus deformity following tibial sesamoidectomy.

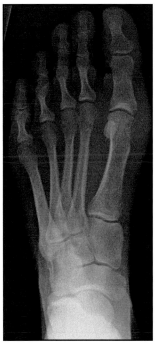

Figure 4-3. Correction following chevron bunionectomy.

trimmed with a saw and a medial capsulorrhaphy is performed after resection of redundant medial capsule. Postoperative management includes a soft bunion dressing with weight bearing as tolerated using a postoperative shoe. The dressing is changed 1 week postoperatively and then discontinued along with the sutures at 2 weeks postoperatively. A removable bunion splint along with a postoperative shoe is then used for an additional 4 weeks. After that, depending on the healing and the patient's residual symptoms, he or she can be transitioned to an accommodative shoe, and gradual return to activity can be implemented. A reasonable estimate for time to return back to running is approximately 3 to 4 months and a time for final outcome is 6 to 12 months postoperatively. In patients who have more severe deformity with an extremely high 1 to 2 intermetatarsal angle, a proximal first metatarsal osteotomy (crescentic or chevron) or a modified Lapidus procedure may be necessary (Figures 4-2 through 4-5).

Suggested Readings

Easley ME, Trnka HJ. Current concepts review: hallux valgus part I: pathomechanics, clinical assessment, and nonoperative management. *Foot Ankle Int.* 2007;28(5):654-659.

Easley ME, Trnka HJ. Current concepts review: hallux valgus part II: operative treatment. *Foot Ankle Int.* 2007;28(6):748-758.

Kelikian AS. Hallux valgus and metatarsus primus varus (HV-MTPV). In: Kelikian AS, ed. *Operative Treatment of the Foot and Ankle.* Stamford, CT: Appleton & Lange; 1999:61-93.

Lillich JS, Baxter DE. Bunionectomies and related surgery in the elite female middle-distance and marathon runner. *Am J Sports Med.* 1986;14(6):491-493.

Figure 4-4. Reduced chevron osteotomy with lateral displacement of metatarsal head and provisional pin fixation at site of absorbable pin placement.

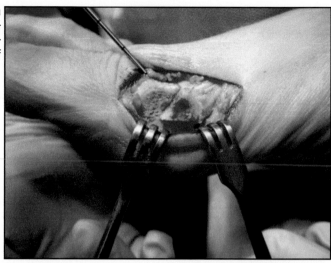

Figure 4-5. Medial capsulorrhaphy repaired.

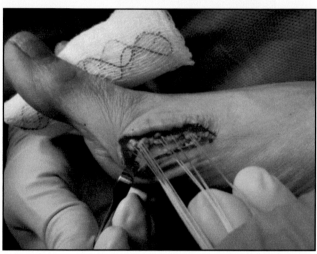

How Would You Treat My 74-Year-Old Community Ambulator With a Severe Bunion Who Cannot Find Shoes for the Michigan Winters?

Robert S. Marsh, DO and Donald R. Bohay, MD, FACS

Hallux valgus has been classified radiographically as mild (hallux valgus angle [HVA] <30 degrees; intermetatarsal angle [IMA] <13 degrees), moderate (HVA = 30 to 40 degrees; IMA = 14 to 20 degrees), and severe (HVA >40 degrees; IMA >20 degrees).[1-3] The primary complaint of a patient with hallux valgus ranges from asymptomatic to painful, debilitating deformity. Unfortunately, even if the deformity is graded as severe but pain free, the one common problem to all types of deformity is the difficulty finding comfortable shoe wear. As the deformity progresses, the foot widens, making standard shoe wear difficult.

Upon the patient's initial presentation to our clinic, we first assess the limits her deformity places on her and perform a targeted physical exam to determine the pathological cause and associated condition that may exist with her deformity. One of the most commonly associated conditions is hypermobility of the first ray associated with gastrocnemius contracture. As the medial column becomes more mobile, it assumes a more extended position. As a result, the patient may experience transfer metatarsalgia as the force from weight bearing is distributed to the lesser metatarsal heads. With time, this can lead to stress fractures of the lesser metatarsal shafts, hammer toe, metatarsalgia, and pes planus.

The first step in the treatment of hallux valgus is patient education as to the nature of the diagnosis. Explaining to the patient why he or she has pain with certain shoes is sometimes difficult. A simple way to display the patient's widened foot is to outline his or her foot on a piece of paper as he or she is standing and compare his or her foot shape to his or her shoe. This often will surprise the patient as to the amount of deformation that occurs to their foot with weight-bearing activities.

Concerning our patient, initial treatment would involve the use of shoes with soft leather uppers and extra width and depth to eliminate the pressure of her widened foot.

If she also is complaining of metatarsalgia, a custom orthotic with a metatarsal pad is often successful in alleviating the metatarsalgia associated with hallux valgus. I have not found that a custom orthotic alone improves the symptoms of hallux valgus. This may be all that is required to keep this 74-year-old community ambulator active and safe throughout the winter.

If she does not respond to conservative treatment, however, I would surgically intervene if she could medically tolerate the procedure. The key here is to assess the nature of her disease. Severe hallux valgus may be associated with advanced osteoarthrosis of the metatarsophalangeal joint. The solution in this case is a metatarsophalangeal joint arthrodesis. I typically use a dorsal incision and, depending on the bone quality, I will use 2 3.5-mm screws in a crossed lag technique, or if the bone is osteopenic, I will add a dorsal plate in compression to provide a more stable construct. With either technique, the patient is placed in a postoperative splint for 2 weeks and then converted to a short leg cast. Typically, she will be partial heel weight bearing for 6 to 8 weeks depending on radiographic signs of union, then she will gradually progress to full weight bearing over the ensuing weeks.

A first tarsometatarsal joint fusion and modified McBride procedure is used if there is hyper mobility of the first ray or if the IMA >15 degrees with relatively nonarthritic metatarsophalangeal joint. I use a dorsal incision with care taken to identify the neurovascular bundle between the first and second metatarsal bases. A transverse arthrotomy is performed at the metatarsocuneiform joint and the cartilage is denuded with a curette. The subchondral bone is then drilled with a 2.0-mm drill, and 2 3.5-mm screws are used to stabilize the joint in the reduced position with care to not plantarflex or dorsiflex the first ray. The first screw starts dorsally on the first metatarsal and runs from a distal-dorsal starting point to engage the plantar medial surface of the medial cuneiform. The second screw starts dorsally just distal to the naviculocuneiform joint and runs from a proximal-dorsal to plantar-distal position, terminating in the base of the first metatarsal (Figure 5-1). In both cases, a burr is used to provide a starting point for the screw to avoid fracture of the bone bridge.

Typically, severe deformities also have an associated contracture of the lateral capsule of the metatarsophalangeal joint and the adductor hallucis. As a result, I routinely perform a modified McBride combined with reefing of the medial capsule to allow a full correction.

Finally, I feel the most important part of any procedure is to correct the gastrocnemius contracture. Correction is performed by using the Silfverskiöld test. With the knee extended, passive dorsiflexion of the ankle is examined and compared to dorsiflexion with the knee flexed. If ankle dorsiflexion does not reach neutral with the knee extended and improves with the knee flexed, a gastrocnemius contracture is present. This is corrected surgically by making a 2-cm longitudinal incision at the juncture of the musculotendinous junction medially. The deep fascia of the leg is exposed and the fascia is entered by using an incision in line with the skin incision. The gastrocnemius aponeurosis is isolated and released transversely with care to only release the tendon and not cut the muscle. Care must be taken to retract and protect the sural nerve on the medial side of the dissection. If the plantaris tendon is found to be contracted as well, it is sharply transected. The foot is then dorsiflexed, resulting in separation of the fascia.

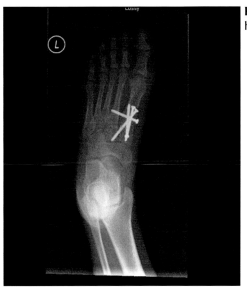

Figure 5-1. Typical screw configuration following hallux valgus correction using a lapidus procedure

Postoperatively, the patient is placed in a well-padded posterior splint and is made nonweight bearing for 6 to 8 weeks depending on radiographic findings. I typically have the patient follow-up 2 weeks following surgery for removal of the splint and sutures, obtain radiographs out of the splint, and place the patient in a cast for 6 additional weeks. At her 8-week postoperative visit, radiographs are again obtained following cast removal and gradual return to full weight bearing is performed over 2 weeks.

References

1. Couglin MJ. Hallux valgus. *J Bone Joint Surg Am*. 1996;78:932-966.
2. Easley ME, Trnka HJ. Current concepts review: hallux valgus part 1: pathomechanics, clinical assessment, and nonoperative management. *Foot Ankle Int*. 2007;28:654-659.
3. Robinson AH, Limbers JP. Modern concepts in the treatment of hallux valgus. *J Bone Joint Surg Br*. 2005;87:1038-1045.

QUESTION

How Do You Treat an Ingrown Toenail? Should I Prescribe the Oral Antifungal Medication for Onychomycosis?

Yong Chae, DPM, FACFAS

How Do You Treat an Ingrown Toenail?

Onychocryptosis of the toenail occurs in all age groups, causing pain and limitation of function. The hallux nail is much more frequently affected than the lesser toes. In patients with mild onychocryptosis or who do not desire surgery, conservative treatment such as soaking in warm water and Epsom salts can be attempted.

Indications for surgery include pain, functional disability, recurrent onychocryptosis, and failure of conservative treatment. Although various procedures are described for treatment of the ingrown nail, I will describe what I consider to be one of the most efficient and successful techniques. The favored procedure in my practice for removal of the ingrown toenail is partial nail avulsion with chemical matrixectomy via application of 89% pure liquefied phenol to the nail bed and underneath the proximal nail fold. I have found that this procedure produces excellent cosmetic and functional results for the patient. Recurrence rates following this procedure are reported to be very low (5%).[1] The procedure can be performed safely in the presence of mild to moderate infection and also in the diabetic patient. Patients with chronically ingrown nails and drainage for 4 weeks should be x-rayed to screen for possible osteomyelitis in the affected digit.[2]

PROCEDURE

A 2-point digital block is administered to the affected toe as follows: Anesthetic is infiltrated from dorsal to plantar on the medial and lateral aspect of the base of the digit. My preferred choice of local anesthetic consists of 1% lidocaine plain and 0.5% bupivacaine plain mixed in a 1:1 ratio. Three mL of the anesthetic is usually sufficient to provide a nerve block for a hallux.

Figure 6-1. Typical instrument tray setup for partial onychoplasty. Instruments from left to right: flat spatula/packer, English anvil nail splitter, #61 blade on Beaver handle, hemostat, small curette, tissue nippers.

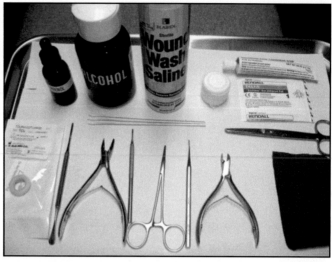

A digital tourniquet is next applied to the base of the toe. This provides a bloodless field for direct visualization of the nail fold and matrix and accurate application of phenol. Excessive bleeding can cause dilution of the phenol, which may result in failure to destroy the matrix. I prefer to use a commercially available prefabricated silicone rubber ring for this purpose. Its benefits include quick and easy application along with exsanguination as it is rolled onto the digit. Alternatively, surgical tubing, Penrose drain tubing, or a finger removed from a latex glove can be used for this purpose. After the tourniquet is applied to the base of the digit and secured with a hemostat, the digit is exsanguinated by slightly pulling on the tubing via the hemostat to allow venous blood flow and by gently squeezing the digit.

The initial approach for a partial matrixectomy is performed with a thin spatula/packer. The thin flat end of the instrument is guided subungually along the border of the affected nail from a distal to proximal direction for the entire length of the nail. Only the portion of the nail that is to be removed should be undermined at this time. It is important to resect enough of the nail plate to alleviate the symptoms, but also to avoid excessive removal of nail for a good cosmetic result. Usually this will be approximately 3 to 4 mm when measured from the nail fold.

The next step involves the use of an English nail splitter (Figure 6-1), which is a specific instrument for accurately splitting the border of the nail that is to be removed. A flat nail nipper can also be used, although caution is required in order to remove only the desired portion of the nail plate. Gentle downward pressure toward the nail bed will help prevent lifting healthy nail off the nail bed.

A small #61 blade is employed to finish the task of nail resection in the most proximal portion of the nail, deep to the proximal nail fold. The blade should be guided carefully to produce a straight incision as an angled incision may lead to a continued painful digit and failure of the matrixectomy. A hemostat is used to grasp the resected nail border, and inward rotation of the instrument toward the nail plate will produce a clean avulsion of the nail border without traumatizing the nail plate (Figure 6-2). A small curette is used to prepare the nail matrix for application of phenol. The nail matrix is gently scraped along the nail bed and also the underside of the proximal nail fold. I routinely attempt

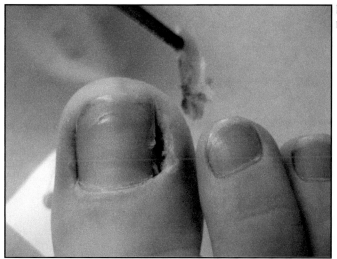

Figure 6-2. Avulsed portion of nail.

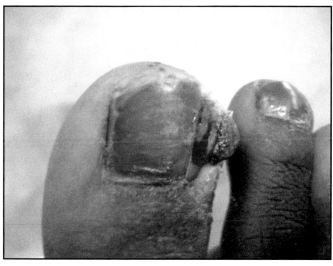

Figure 6-3. Granulomatous tissue of the lateral nail border. This can be easily resected with tissue nippers.

to directly visualize the most proximal portion of the resected nail to ensure that no nail spicules remain.

After removal of the ingrown toenail, hypertrophic nail fold or granulomatous tissue should be resected with tissue nippers. The hypertrophic tissues are cleared from the eponychium to the distal end of the toe. If the hypertrophic tissue is not resected, it can continue to cause symptoms of the ingrown nail along with permanent enlargement of the affected side of the toe (Figure 6-3).

Phenol is then applied to the nail border for destruction of the nail matrix. I will use micro-tip cotton-tipped applicators for this purpose; however, regular-sized cotton-tipped applicators with the excess cotton removed and fashioned into small points can be used as well. The applicators are dipped into the phenol and then gauze is used to soak away the excess. Extreme care must be employed when handling phenol as it is very caustic. Three applicators are applied for approximately 30 seconds each. Proper destruction of the nail matrix is heralded by the whitish blanched appearance of the nail bed after

Figure 6-4. Final appearance of nail border after avulsion of nail and application of phenol. Note the blanched appearance of the nail bed/matrix.

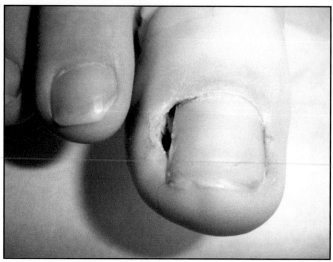

phenolization (Figure 6-4). I then immediately flush the nail fold with isopropyl alcohol and follow with normal saline for a final irrigation of the site. The wound is packed with Bacitracin ointment and then wrapped with a nonstick dressing, 1″ roll gauze, and cohesive bandage as a final layer. The tourniquet is finally removed. This procedure generally takes 5 minutes to complete.

Postoperative course consists of 5- to 10-minute daily soaks in weak Epsom salts and lukewarm water followed by application of Bacitracin ointment. I also prescribe Cortisporin Otic Solution (neomycin, polymyxin sulfates, and hydrocortisone otic solution) in cases of excessive drainage and continued inflammation. I recommend this for 1 to 2 weeks as long as the wound is draining. Total healing times can vary from 2 to 5 weeks.

Potential complications can include regrowth of the nail, nail deformity secondary to over application of phenol and subsequent damage to healthy nail, continued paronychia, and pain due to insufficient nail margin excision. Overapplication of phenol can also result in prolonged drainage, tissue slough, and periostitis.

Should I Prescribe the Oral Antifungal Medication for Onychomycosis?

Onychomycosis is the most common nail disease, accounting for about half of nail pathologies.[3] If untreated, it can lead to pain, discomfort in shoes, infection, and subungual ulceration. There may also be increased self-consciousness of the disfigured nails, which can have psychosocial and emotional effects.[4] Diabetic patients are at increased risk of infectious complications.

Diagnosis of onychomycosis is generally made based on its typical clinical appearance. When the diagnosis is in doubt, I recommend laboratory testing with potassium hydroxide preparation and also periodic acid Schiff testing of the nail.

Treatment of onychomycosis can consist of topical or oral antifungal medications. In general, topical agents such as ciclopirox olamine 8% should be used as monotherapy only in cases involving less than half of the distal nail plate. Although topical agents improve the cure rate and shorten the duration of treatment when used alongside oral antifungal therapy, they are rarely sufficient when used as monotherapy. Patients treated with oral antifungal therapy for onychomycosis report significantly higher satisfaction and clinical improvement than patients treated with topical therapy.[5]

Currently, terbinafine (Lamisil) and itraconazole (Sporanox) are US Food and Drug Administration approved for the treatment of onychomycosis. The reported mycological cure rates are higher for terbinafine compared with itraconazole.[6]

The adult dose of terbinafine for toenail infection is 250 mg daily for 12 weeks. It can also be pulsed dosed at 500 mg daily for 1 week every month for 4 months. My preference is for daily dosing as I have observed higher success rates and patient compliance with this regimen.

Common adverse effects of the medication can include headache, diarrhea, dyspepsia, taste disturbance, and vision changes. Mild rash, pruritus, urticaria, toxic epidermal necrolysis, and erythema multiforme have also been reported. Rarely, liver injury has also been reported as well.[6] In my experience, gastrointestinal symptoms were most frequent and resolved with discontinuation of the medication.

The approved dosage of itraconazole is 200 mg once daily for 12 weeks. I have also treated patients with pulse dosing as well, which consists of 400 mg daily for 1 week every month for 3 months. While itraconazole is effective for the treatment of onychomycosis, it has a much more extensive list of drug interactions than terbinafine and can cause serious toxicity when taken with other drugs metabolized by the cytochrome P450 isoenzymes.

I routinely perform a baseline liver function panel prior to initiating oral therapy. I also follow up with a 6-week liver function panel. I have observed very little if any change in transaminase levels with terbinafine. Therefore, with the well-established safety profile of terbinafine, high success rates, and overall patient satisfaction, I consider oral antifungal therapy the treatment of choice for onychomycosis.

References

1. Salasche SJ. Surgery. In: Scher RK, Daniel CR, eds. *Nails: Therapy, Diagnosis, Surgery*. Philadelphia, PA: WB Saunders; 2005:326-349.
2. Cox HA, Jones RO. Direct extension osteomyelitis secondary to chronic onychocryptosis. Three case reports *J Am Podiatric Med Assoc*. 1995;85:321-324.
3. Szepietowski JC, Salomon J. Do fungi play a role in psoriatic nails? *Mycoses*. 2007;50(6):437-442.
4. Lubeck DP. Measuring health-related quality of life in onychomycosis. *J Am Acad Dermatol*. 1998;38(5 Pt 3):S64-S68.
5. Stier D. Patient satisfaction with oral versus nonoral therapeutic approaches in onychomycosis. *J Am Podiatric Med Assoc*. 2001;91:521-527.
6. Terbinafine for onychomycosis. *Med Lett*. 1996;38:72-74.

How Do You Manage Hallux Rigidus? Which Patients With Hallux Rigidus Should Receive a Cheilectomy, Arthrodesis, or Arthroplasty?

Jennifer Chu, MD and Judith Baumhauer, MD, MPH

Hallux rigidus is a spectrum of degenerative arthritis of the first metatarsophalangeal (MTP) joint and is characterized by periarticular osteophyte formation and restricted motion, particularly dorsiflexion. Patients present with pain localized to the first MTP joint. On physical exam, joint tenderness, swelling, and restricted motion may be seen. Radiographs will show first MTP joint space narrowing and marginal osteophytes.[1] A dorsal first metatarsal osteophyte may be seen on a lateral view. A grading system based on range of motion, radiographs, and clinical exam has been developed for hallux rigidus (Table 7-1).[2]

When a patient initially presents to the clinic with hallux rigidus, I will prescribe a Morton's extension carbon foot plate with mild stiffness (Figure 7-1). I explain to patients that this orthosis may alleviate their pain by decreasing motion across the first MTP joint. I also recommend shoe wear modifications, including choosing footwear with a wide toe box to decrease pressure on the dorsal bony prominence and a stiffer sole. I will suggest nonsteroidal anti-inflammatory drugs as needed.[3]

If the patient continues to have pain after a trial of nonoperative management, I will consider surgical management. My first-line surgical treatment in patients with Grade 1 or 2 disease and isolated dorsal great toe pain and without inflammatory arthritis is a cheilectomy. When explaining surgery to patients, I will show them their lateral foot radiograph and point out the dorsal metatarsal head osteophyte that I will be resecting (Figure 7-2). I am careful to tell patients that this procedure does not cure arthritis but may decrease pain by decreasing the bony impingement of the osteophytes. This surgery burns no bridges, and other procedures can be performed at a later date should pain persist. One major reason for failure of a cheilectomy is inadequate bone resection, which will lead to persistent impingement of the proximal phalanx against the metatarsal head dorsal osteophyte. The dorsal one-third of the metatarsal head and all osteophytes should

<u>Table 7-1</u>

Radiographic System for Grading Hallux Rigidus

Grade	Dorsiflexion	Radiographic Findings*	Clinical Findings
0	40 to 60 degrees and/or 10% to 20% loss compared with normal side	Normal	No pain; only stiffness and loss of motion on examination
1	30 to 40 degrees and/or 20% to 50% loss compared with normal side	Dorsal osteophyte is main finding, minimal joint space narrowing, minimal periarticular sclerosis, minimal flattening of metatarsal head	Mild or occasional pain and stiffness; pain at extremes of dorsiflexion and/or plantarflexion on examination
2	10 to 30 degrees and/or 50% to 75% loss compared with normal side	Dorsal, lateral, and possibly medial osteophytes giving flattened appearance to metatarsal head, no more than 1/4 of dorsal joint space involved on lateral radiograph, mild to moderate joint space narrowing and sclerosis, sesamoids not usually involved	Moderate to severe pain and stiffness that may be constant; pain occurs just before maximum dorsiflexion and maximum plantarflexion on examination
3	≤10 degrees and/or 75% to 100% loss compared with normal side. There is notable loss of MTP plantarflexion as well (often ≤10 degrees of plantarflexion)	Same as in Grade 2 but with substantial narrowing, possibly periarticular cystic changes, more than 1/4 of dorsal joint space involved on lateral radiograph, sesamoids enlarged and/or cystic and/or irregular	Nearly constant pain and substantial stiffness at extremes of range of motion but not at mid-range
4	Same as in Grade 3	Same as in Grade 3	Same as in Grade 3 but there is definite pain at mid-range of passive motion

*Weight-bearing and anteroposterior and lateral radiographs are used.

Reprinted with permission from Coughlin M, Shurnas P. Hallux rigidus: grading and long term results of operative treatment. *J Bone Joint Surg Am.* 2003;85(11):2072-2088.

be removed. Only 11 degrees of improved motion is achieved with a cheilectomy, so I make sure my patients understand that this surgery will not significantly increase the motion at this joint.

I advocate arthrodesis for patients with known inflammatory arthritis or dorsal and plantar great toe pain. This will provide reliable pain relief at the first MTP joint at the expense of motion. Patients will be unable to wear shoes with a heel height greater than 1 to 2 inches. Often, patients who are good candidates for arthrodesis already have motion limitations preoperatively, so it is easy for them to understand what their

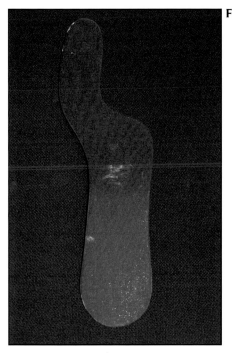

Figure 7-1. Carbon foot plate.

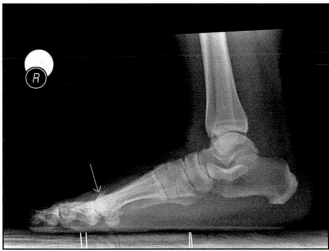

Figure 7-2. Lateral foot radiograph of a patient who later underwent cheilectomy. The white arrow points to the dorsal osteophyte.

limitations will be postoperatively. Several options including plate and screw constructs, compression screws, or threaded Steinmann pins achieve fusion, and each of these has been shown to have high success rates. I use a lag screw and plate construct because this has been found biomechanically superior to crossed lag screws. The great toe should be placed in 25 degrees of dorsiflexion in relation to the first metatarsal declination angle and slight valgus so the toe lies next to the second toe. After the procedure, I will keep patients nonweight bearing for 1 to 2 weeks for wound healing. Patients are placed in a walking boot and I allow them to weight bear as tolerated. I usually keep patients in a walking boot for 4 weeks. Potential complications of arthrodesis include malunion, nonunion, and hallux interphalangeal joint degenerative arthritis, which has been linked to inadequate positioning of the toe in neutral or varus.

At this time, I do not use implant arthroplasty for the treatment of hallux rigidus. Intermediate and long-term studies of previous implant models, including silicone elastomer implants and metal-polyethylene joint replacements, show high rates of failure and inconsistent pain relief. There are increased complications of arthroplasty when compared to arthrodesis. One of my greatest concerns with arthroplasty is the amount of bone resection required, which can complicate revision or salvage procedures. The shortened first ray can result in transfer metatarsalgia and require arthrodesis with structural bone graft for salvage.

References

1. Shurnas P. Hallux rigidus. In: Pinzur M, ed. *Orthopaedic Knowledge Update: Foot and Ankle*. Rosemont, IL: American Academy of Orthopaedic Surgeons; 2008:249-255.
2. Coughlin M, Shurnas P. Hallux rigidus: grading and long term results of operative treatment. *J Bone Joint Surg Am*. 2003;85(11):2072-2088.
3. Colman A, Pomeroy G. First metatarsophalangeal disorders. In: DiGiovanni C, Greisberg J, eds. *Foot and Ankle: Core Knowledge in Orthopaedics*. Philadelphia, PA: Elsevier Mosby; 2007:119-124.

How Do I Perform a Midfoot Fusion?

Michael S. Pinzur, MD

The tarsometatarsal (TMT) junction is a unique functional entity. While there is a minimal amount of motion during the transition from midstance to push-off, this critical joint appears to very efficiently transmit the load of weight bearing.[1] Patients rarely recover full function following injury to this crucial joint.[2] Once we appreciate this complex nature of this crucial joint, we are more likely to perform arthrodesis only after we have failed at accommodative therapy.

My initial recommendation for treatment of TMT arthritis is accommodative orthotic management. My "blue-plate special" is an oxford tie shoe with a cushioned heel to absorb the impact of initial loading (ie, heel strike) and a rocker sole to simulate the motion and decrease the load on the tarsal metatarsal junction during the critical terminal period of stance phase. I also use fluoroscopic-guided steroid injections. When steroid injections and therapeutic accommodation are unsuccessful, I then recommend arthrodesis. I often combine local anesthetics with the steroid to determine if the lateral joints will require arthrodesis of the third TMT joint or interpositional arthroplasty of the fourth and fifth TMT joints.

During terminal stance phase, the first, second, and third TMT joints are sequentially loaded, forming the so-called stable medial column. The final period of stance is associated with motion in the fourth and fifth TMT joints.[1] Therefore, my first step is arthrodesis of the first and second TMT joints through a single dorsal incision. When the third TMT joint is involved, I perform the arthrodesis of that joint through a second dorsal incision. The final step, when necessary, is an interpositional arthroplasty of the fourth and fifth TMT joints through this same incision.

I will generally use a small narrow oscillating power saw to prepare the joint surfaces for the arthrodesis. This method creates a cabinetmaker's dovetailed joint as well as allows the forefoot to be appropriately plantarflexed. If there is bone loss, I have a very low threshold to restore medial column length with a trapezoidal-shaped tricortical autologous iliac crest bone graft. My bias is to use a screw-plate construct to perform the first and second TMT fusion as opposed to crossed screws. Several of the device

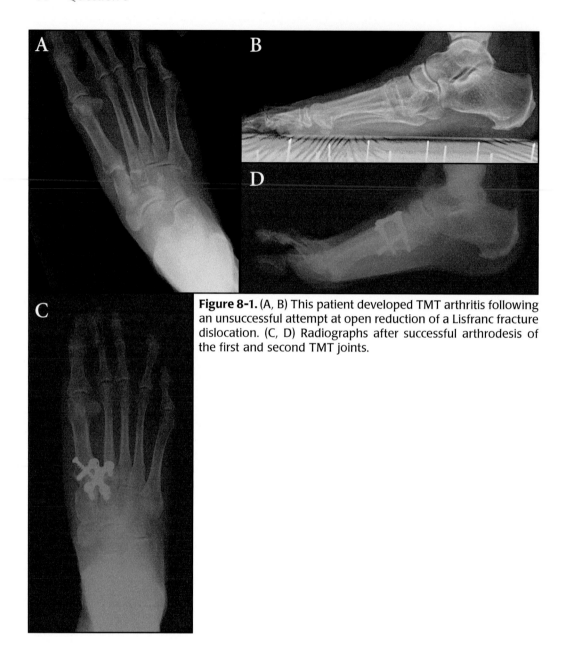

Figure 8-1. (A, B) This patient developed TMT arthritis following an unsuccessful attempt at open reduction of a Lisfranc fracture dislocation. (C, D) Radiographs after successful arthrodesis of the first and second TMT joints.

manufacturers now have dorsal plates that are specifically designed for this application (Figure 8-1). In order to obtain stable fixation, I also have a reasonably low threshold to span joints not included in the arthrodesis. Following successful arthrodesis, many of these screws will fracture, or the dorsal plates will fracture over the mobile joint, making hardware removal unnecessary.

My current personal preference is to inject 2 ccs of bone marrow aspirate and one syringe of autologous platelet-rich concentrate to augment bony healing. When recombinant growth factors become commercially available, I plan to continue the practice of adding the pluripotential stem cells derived from the one marrow aspirate, but substitute the autologous platelet-rich concentrate with growth factor.

If the wound appears secure at the first postoperative visit, I apply a short leg walking cast or a fracture boot in reliable patients and allow weight bearing as tolerated.

References

1. Lakin RC, DeGnore LT, Pienkowski D. Contact mechanics of normal tarsometatarsal joints. *J Bone Joint Surg.* 2001;83A:520-528.
2. Teng A, Pinzur MS, Lomasney L, Mahoney L, Havey R. Functional outcome following anatomic restoration of tarsal-metatarsal fracture dislocation. *Foot Ankle Int.* 2002;23:922-926.

SECTION II

HINDFOOT

QUESTION

9

How Do You Treat Plantar Fasciitis? How Do I Know if It Is the First Branch of the Lateral Plantar Nerve (Baxter's Nerve)?

Bruce Cohen, MD

There are many things to consider when assessing a patient with heel pain. The location of the pain is critical in determining both the pathology and the treatment options. Posterior heel pain is typically related to Achilles tendon insertional pathology. Central heel pad-type pain may be related to insufficiency of the heel pad or may be the result of neuritis of the first branch of the lateral plantar nerve. The classic presentation of plantar fasciitis is pain at the origin of the plantar fascia, typically along the medial cord. The patient typically complains of pain with the first step in the morning or when rising from a seated position. The pain is relieved with rest and often improves with further activity. We will discuss the treatment options for plantar fasciitis as well as the differentiation of the classic plantar fasciitis versus neuritis of the first branch of the lateral plantar nerve, often described as Baxter's nerve.

The challenge in treating heel pain is differentiating between the classic plantar fasciitis and the neuritis of the first branch of the lateral plantar nerve. Baxter originally described this entity in 1992 as a cause of chronic heel pain in active patients.[1] The symptoms are different from the classic plantar fasciitis. The history is critical in treating this patient. Patients complain of a burning-type pain that continues even when they get off their feet. We commonly call this an "after-burn." This pain can wake them from sleep and occurs with both weight bearing and nonweight bearing. On physical examination, the patient can have plantar medial heel pain but the tenderness is more commonly maximized over the abductor hallucis region medially. There may be proximal radiation and even a Tinel's sign on occasion. Many patients describe a change in their symptoms over time, especially in the face of repeated corticosteroid injections.[2] In this scenario, initial symptoms of plantar fasciitis are replaced with more proximal neuritic pain as described above. The diagnostic workup has not been very helpful. Magnetic resonance imaging typically is not beneficial, with the most common findings being consistent with chronic plantar fasciitis. Nerve conduction studies and electromyography are typically normal. This diagnosis is clinical and can be made based on correlation of the physical exam findings and the pertinent characteristics of the pain on history.[3]

The treatments of plantar fasciitis and neuritis of the first branch of the lateral plantar nerve, which we will term *distal tarsal tunnel syndrome*, are different. The mainstay of treatment of plantar fasciitis is conservative. The treatment can be divided into the following 4 stages:

1. Stage 1 consists of home-directed plantar fascial and Achilles stretching, over-the-counter nonsteroidal anti-inflammatory drugs (NSAIDs), and off-the-shelf orthotic devices. Digiovanni et al described a plantar-fascial specific stretching program with excellent results.[4] I will often use over-the-counter cushioned arch supports rather than heel cushions alone to provide better longitudinal arch support. The use of a dorsiflexion night splint is considered in this stage.

2. Stage 2 consists of supervised physical therapy and modalities such as ultrasound and iontophoresis. In this stage, I will frequently prescribe custom orthotic devices. A trial of prescription NSAIDs is also reasonable.

3. Stage 3 is typically a period of immobilization. I prefer a short leg walking cast for 4 weeks but occasionally will use a removable boot for a similar time period.

4. Stage 4 is considered a failure of conservative management and I will recommend high-energy extracorporeal shockwave therapy or surgical release of the medial band of the plantar fascia. My preference is the shockwave treatment versus surgery, but insurance oftentimes does not cover this treatment modality and surgery is recommended.

When treating distal tarsal tunnel syndrome, I will still use Stages 1 through 3 but will not typically recommend shockwave treatment. If surgery is recommended, it includes a partial plantar fascial release and a distal tarsal tunnel release including the lateral plantar nerve and infrequently the medial plantar nerve.[5]

The surgical technique for the release of the first branch of the lateral plantar nerve and the distal tarsal tunnel is performed through regional anesthesia by popliteal block or general anesthesia. An incision is made extending from the proximal edge of the flexor retinaculum and extended plantar and distal to the inferior border of the abductor hallucis fascia. When combining with a partial plantar fascial release, which is commonly performed in my practice, the incision is extended across the proximal portion of the plantar skin at the origin of the plantar fascia (Figure 9-1). The flexor retinaculum is released and the deep and superficial investing fascia of the abductor hallucis is released (Figures 9-2 and 9-3). Care should be taken to preserve the muscle fibers to prevent bleeding and scar tissue formation. The nerve is underlying the deep fascia and neurolysis should be avoided. A release of all fascial bands should be performed, including the fascia of the quadratus plantae. When addressing compression of the medial plantar nerve as well, the separate fascial tunnel through the abductor should be released. When combining with a plantar fascial release, the medial 50% of the plantar fascia is released. The postoperative course includes an immediate nonweight-bearing splint for 10 to 14 days followed by a boot. Weight bearing is allowed at 3 weeks postoperatively and range of motion is allowed at the first postoperative visit. The boot is typically discontinued at 6 weeks.

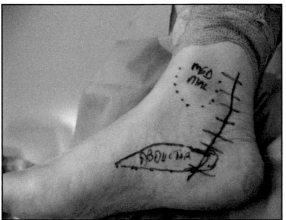

Figure 9-1. Incision for distal tarsal tunnel release.

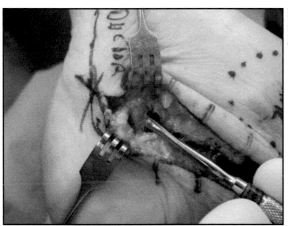

Figure 9-2. The flexor retinaculum is released and the superficial fascia of the abductor is being shown.

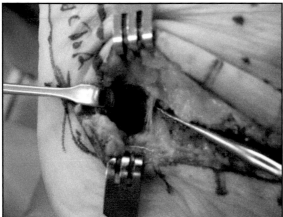

Figure 9-3. The superficial and fascia of the abductor hallucis is released and the deep fascia is shown. The lateral plantar nerve lies directly beneath this layer.

References

1. Baxter DE. Pfeffer GB. Treatment of chronic heel pain by surgical release of the first branch of the lateral plantar nerve. *Clin Orthop.* 1992;(279):229-236.
2. Acevedo JI, Beskin JL. Complications of plantar fascia rupture associated with corticosteroid injection. *Foot Ankle Int.* 1998;19(2):91-97.
3. Cimino WR. Tarsal tunnel syndrome: review of the literature. *Foot Ankle.* 1990;11(1):47-52.
4. Digiovanni BF, Nawoszenski DA, Malay DP, et al. Plantar fascia-specific stretching exercise improves outcomes in patients with chronic plantar fasciitis. A prospective clinical trial with two-year follow-up. *J Bone Joint Surg Am.* 2006;88(8):1775-1781.
5. Labib SA, Gould JS, Rodriguez-del-Rio FA, Lyman S. Heel pain triad (HPT): the combination of plantar fasciitis, posterior tibial tendon dysfunction and tarsal tunnel syndrome. *Foot Ankle Int.* 2002;23(3):212-220.

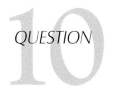
DO ALL PATIENTS WITH PES PLANUS REQUIRE TREATMENT?

Eric Breitbart, MD; Wayne Berberian, MD; and Sheldon Lin, MD

For the purpose of this discussion, I will be focusing on adult-acquired flatfoot deformity (AAFD), also known as posterior tibial tendon dysfunction. The way I approach my patients with AAFD is based upon an individualized plan depending on his or her symptomatology, history, and most importantly, the stage of the deformity. Stage of deformity is a uniform way to select your treatment plan. AAFD has been classified into 4 stages, with Johnson and Strom describing Stages I through III, and Myerson adding a Stage IV.[1] Stage I consists of painful tenosynovitis of the posterior tibial tendon; however, the tendon itself is of normal length and function and has no visible deformity. Stage II consists of a flatfoot deformity with pain and dysfunction of the posterior tibial tendon. Patients have normal hindfoot motion but are unable to perform a single-leg heel rise. Stage III, like the earlier stages, also includes dysfunction of the posterior tibial tendon; however, the hindfoot joints are stiff and arthritic. Stage IV consists of a Stage III deformity with additional evidence of associated tibiotalar asymmetry because of the prolonged hindfoot valgus deformity.

In terms of treatment, I divide my patients into flexible (Stage I and II) and rigid (Stage III and IV) AAFD. For patients with a flexible deformity, I recommend conservative nonsurgical treatment. Nonsurgical management focuses on improving a patient's symptoms by decreasing the forces going through the posteromedial hindfoot.[2] First, starting patients on a course of a nonsteroidal anti-inflammatory medication may help with some mild pain relief. Patients with Stage I or II AAFD may be immobilized with a short leg cast or controlled ankle motion walker and production of a custom orthosis (ie, University of California Berkley orthosis) with the hindfoot casted in neutral position. In my symptomatic patients with a flexible flatfoot, I will place them in a custom-molded ankle-foot orthosis, such as an Arizona AFO (Arizona AFO, Inc, Mesa, AZ), in order to increase stability of the ankle. In addition to bracing or casting in a relatively asymptomatic patient, stabilization/improvement of the disease can be achieved through weight loss and activity modification. While not used routinely in my practice, recent protocol modification also discusses the role of physical therapy and specific exercise regimens.[3]

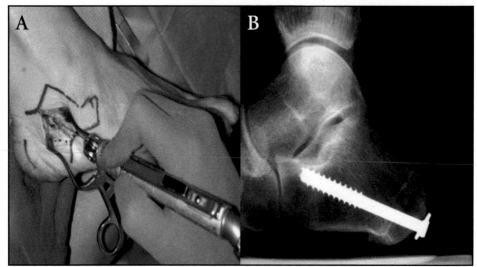

Figure 10-1. Posterior tibial tendon reconstruction with medial calcaneal osteotomy. (A) Note the lateral incision posterior to the peroneal tendons with a transverse osteotomy being performed of the calcaneal tubercle. (B) The osteotomy is subsequently fixed with a single partially threaded screw through the calcaneus from posterior to anterior.

Before I consider nonsurgical management to be a failure, I usually wait to see whether symptoms worsen in spite of bracing or if improvements fail to be observed in the patient's pain/functioning in 4 to 6 months. If conservative therapy does fail, a wide array of surgical options are available. Prior to considering surgery in any of my patients, their risk factor for poor outcomes must be assessed. These risk factors include smoking, uncontrolled diabetes mellitus, chronic steroid use, and a history of noncompliance with treatment regimens. Patients with one or more of these risk factors should have the risk factors optimized prior to surgical intervention.

In the rare case in which a patient with Stage I AAFD fails to be helped by conservative therapy, I have noticed that tenosynovectomy of the posterior tibial tendon has provided significant reduction in pain in some of my patients. Out of all the AAFD stages, Stage II has the widest array of surgical options depending on the degree of deformity. My surgery of choice is the posterior tibial tendon reconstruction, flexor digitorum longus (FDL) transfer with a medial slide calcaneal osteotomy, especially if a valgus deformity is present in the hindfoot (Figure 10-1).[4] Variations of this procedure include adding a spring ligament repair, advancing the FDL insertion (such as the FDL into the medial cuneiform) for the repair and adding a procedure like triple hemiresection method of Hoke or gastrocnemius recession to correct an equinus contracture if one exists.

In the presence of significant forefoot abduction, surgical options for Stage II AAFD may involve lateral column lengthening with or without calcaneal osteotomies (Figure 10-2). Lengthening the lateral column corrects the deformity by adducting and plantarflexing the midfoot around the talar head. However, complications with this procedure can be relatively high, including abnormal gait (forefoot varus with the patient walking on the lateral border of his or her foot), lateral overload, graft failure, nonunion of the structural graft, and painful hardware, hence my reluctance to use it.[5]

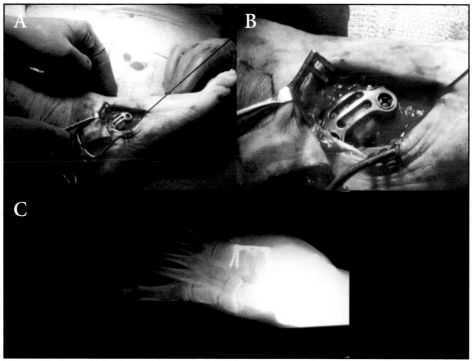

Figure 10-2. Lateral column lengthening of the calcaneocuboid joint. (A, B) Intraoperative photos showing a successfully implanted graft between the calcaneus and cuboid fixed using a cervical plate. (C) Anteroposterior radiograph of the ankle postoperatively demonstrating proper alignment of the graft.

Surgery is almost always necessary in order to improve pain and function in a rigid hindfoot patient. While you should always give a brief trial of conservative therapy, including weight loss, activity modification, and casting/bracing, with a rigid flatfoot deformity, patients are counseled on its poor success. These patients have hindfoot joints that are arthritic and would not benefit from any nonoperative treatments, but rather require arthrodesis. If only the joints of the hindfoot are involved, I would approach these patients with the gold standard surgical management of a triple arthrodesis. If the tibiotalar joint is also involved (as in Stage IV AAFD), I would change this procedure to a tibiotalocalcaneal arthrodesis. I typically reserve arthrodesis for only those with Stage III and IV AAFD (those who already have evidence of arthritis) because hindfoot arthrodesis limits motion and forces the remaining joints to absorb a greater amount of force. I always warn my patients that because of these changes in force distribution, an arthrodesis has a significant risk of contiguous joint arthritis in the future.

Conclusion

In my practice I generally approach Stage I and II AAFD with conservative management first, and if the patient is dissatisfied, this practice is followed by hindfoot motion-sparing procedures. In Stage III and IV AAFD, because of underlying degenerative joint disease in the hindfoot, arthrodesis is necessary for relief of symptomatology and correction of the deformity.

References

1. Myerson MS, Corrigan J. Treatment of posterior tibial tendon dysfunction with flexor digitorum longus tendon transfer and calcaneal osteotomy. *Orthopedics.* 1996;19(5):383-388.
2. Lin JL, Balbas J, Richardson EG. Results of non-surgical treatment of stage II posterior tibial tendon dysfunction: a 7- to 10-year followup. *Foot Ankle Int.* 2008;29(8):781-786.
3. Alvarez RG, Marini A, Schmitt C, Saltzman CL. Stage I and II posterior tibial tendon dysfunction treated by a structured nonoperative management protocol: an orthosis and exercise program. *Foot Ankle Int.* 2006;27(1):2-8.
4. Myerson MS, Badekas A, Schon LC. Treatment of stage II posterior tibial tendon deficiency with flexor digitorum longus tendon transfer and calcaneal osteotomy. *Foot Ankle Int.* 2004;25(7):445-450.
5. Toolan BC, Sangeorzan BJ, Hansen ST Jr. Complex reconstruction for the treatment of dorsolateral peritalar subluxation of the foot. Early results after distraction arthrodesis of the calcaneocuboid joint in conjunction with stabilization of, and transfer of the flexor digitorum longus tendon to, the midfoot to treat acquired pes planovalgus in adults. *J Bone Joint Surg Am.* 1999;81(11):1545-1560.

WHAT IS YOUR SURGICAL APPROACH TO CHRONIC POSTERIOR TIBIAL TENDON INSUFFICIENCY?

Scott Nemec, DO and John G. Anderson, MD

When dealing with posterior tibial tendon pathology, the pathologic reason for the problem must be understood. There are many variations of arch collapse, with multiple components to each flatfoot deformity. Arch collapse is the result of a breakdown in the medial column-supporting structures of the longitudinal and transverse arch. This includes the plantar fascia, short and long plantar ligaments, capsular ligaments, spring ligament, and posterior tibial tendon. This collapse can be aggravated or precipitated by several factors, including body weight, female sex, trauma, and medical conditions such as diabetes and rheumatoid arthritis, among others. Equinus contracture is a common factor in the far majority of these deformities.

As the foot progresses to the acquired flatfoot deformity, breakdown of the medial column results. The equinus contracture pulls the calcaneus into relative plantarflexion. The talus follows and eventually plantarflexes as it rotates through the subtalar joint. This results in a lateral peritalar subluxation as the spring ligament becomes attenuated and ground reaction force drives the forefoot into relative dorsiflexion, or varus. A varus forefoot results, with a midfoot that drifts into abduction (Figures 11-1 and 11-2). The hindfoot falls into increasing valgus. The tibialis posterior and spring ligament eventually fail and the resulting flatfoot deformity becomes irreversible.

Treatment must take into account the reason that the foot has assumed the flatfoot deformity and must accommodate all aspects of the deformity. The equinus driving force must be addressed while also correcting associated forefoot varus, hindfoot valgus, posterior tibial tendon disruption, or existing arthritic joints. A gastrocnemius recession is used to address the equinus deformity. This helps to unload the forefoot and repositions the hindfoot out of equinus, which helps facilitate the correction of any forefoot or hindfoot deformity during subsequent corrective procedures. Additional bony and soft tissue procedures are necessary to address the forefoot varus and hindfoot valgus. A medializing calcaneal osteotomy is performed to address the valgus hindfoot alignment (Figure 11-3). If there is uncoverage greater than 30% at the talonavicular joint as a

Figure 11-1. Dorsolateral peritalar subluxation is seen, with resulting increased abduction of the forefoot and talonavicular uncoverage. Functionally short lateral column is seen.

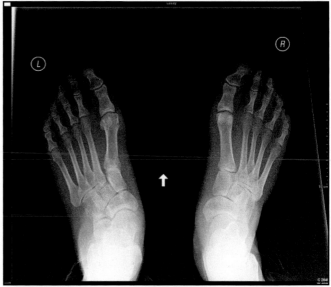

Figure 11-2. Relative plantarflexion of the calcaneus and talus are seen in the weight-bearing image. Loss of medial column height is noted as medial cuneiform is superimposed on fifth metatarsal. Accessory navicular is also present.

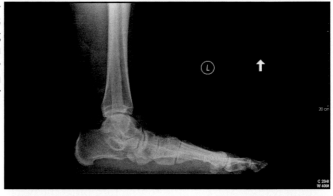

Figure 11-3. Medializing calcaneal osteotomy correcting hindfoot valgus alignment.

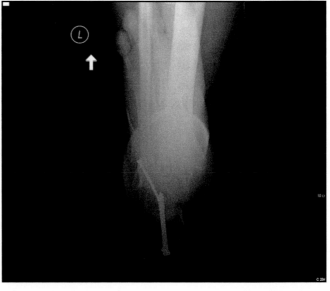

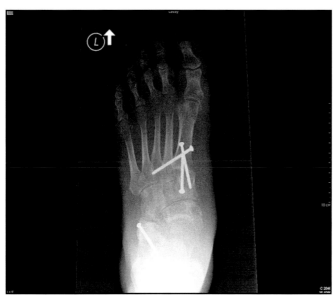

Figure 11-4. After reconstruction. Note lateral column lengthening fixation and fusion of the medial column. The talonavicular joint is reduced with complete coverage after lateral column procedure. Bony tunnel in the navicular is seen where flexor digitorum longus (FDL) transfer occurred.

result of the dorsolateral peritalar subluxation, a lateral column-lengthening procedure is also used to correct the functionally short lateral column. This will essentially push the forefoot out of abduction and cover the talus at the talonavicular joint. This procedure is performed through the utilization of a standard lateral longitudinal approach to the sinus tarsi. The anterior process of the calcaneus is identified and cut just distal to the crucial angle. Lamina spreaders are used to lengthen the lateral column. Upon determining the necessary amount of distraction, an allograft tricortical iliac crest bone graft is fashioned and placed into the osteotomy site. The medial column incompetence is then addressed by performing a medial column fusion, such as a first tarsometatarsal arthrodesis, naviculocuneiform arthrodesis, or a combination of both. Additional coronal plane deformity of the first ray is corrected through a Lapidus-type reconstruction, which stabilizes for medial column collapse and corrects forefoot varus while simultaneously correcting the hallux valgus and metatarsus primus varus. Residual motion in the sagittal plane is often encountered through the intercuneiform joint, which is addressed with an intermetatarsal arthrodesis between the first and second metatarsals (Figures 11-4 and 11-5). The posterior tibialis tendon is then inspected through a standard medial incision. Inspection of the spring ligament also occurs at this time. If the spring ligament is torn, it should be débrided and repaired. In scenarios where the tendon demonstrates degenerative change or longitudinal tearing but has maintained excursion, the tendon is débrided and repaired. The flexor digitorum longus (FDL) tendon is identified and harvested and transferred to the posterior tibialis tendon to aid in function. This may be done with a side-to-side repair technique or a Pulvertaft weave-type procedure. In cases where the tibialis posterior tendon demonstrates lack of motion, the tendon is excised completely. In this situation, the FDL tendon is transferred to either the navicular or the medial cuneiform via bony tunnels. Diligence must must be used to ensure that enough FDL graft is harvested. Dissection must be taken distally past the master knot of Henry to free enough tendon to ensure adequate length for transfer. Upon completing this, the components of the flatfoot deformity have been corrected, thus restoring plantigrade alignment to the

Figure 11-5. After reconstruction, the calcaneal osteotomy and lateral column lengthening solidly healed. Medial column fused restoring stability. Note the restored alignment of the talo-metatarsal line, along with the restored medial column height. Accessory navicular has been excised.

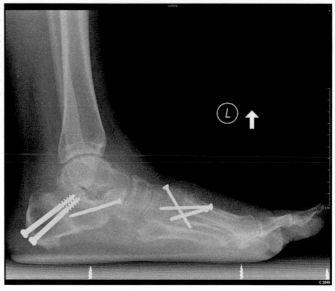

foot. Postoperative care includes 2 weeks in a bulky splint, followed by removal of sutures and placement into a short leg cast. Weight bearing is delayed for 8 weeks, followed by progressive weight-bearing as tolerated in a removable boot. Standard shoe wear is usually achievable at 3 months.

Suggested Readings

Anderson JG, Hansen ST. Surgical treatment of posterior tibial tendon pathology. In: Kelikian AS, ed. *Operative Treatment of the Foot and Ankle*. Stamford, CT: Appleton and Lange; 1999:211-231.

Mosier-LaClair S, Pomeroy G, Manoli A 2nd. Operative treatment of the difficult stage 2 adult acquired flatfoot deformity. *Foot Ankle Clin*. 2001;6(1):95-119.

Sands AK, Tansey JP. Lateral column lengthening. *Foot Ankle Clin*. 2007;12(2):301-308, vi-vii.

WHICH PATIENTS WITH CAVOVARUS FEET NEED TREATMENT?

Armen S. Kelikian, MD

I believe all patients with cavovarus feet need treatment; the only question is determining the level of treatment required. There are numerous etiologies that have been reported, but I will discuss the most commonly encountered ones. Once the etiology has been determined, treatment can begin. Twenty-three percent of the population has cavovarus and the majority of these are idiopathic in the adult population. Charcot-Marie-Tooth is common in the pediatric setting. It is usually autosomal dominant (Type I-A & B, II) but can be recessive (IV) or X-linked as well. There are numerous other conditions in the differential such as Friedreich's ataxia, cerebral palsy, and syringomyelia.[1]

There is a wide variety of clinical presentation. Ankle instability, arthritis, lateral foot or ankle pain, and first ray metatarsalgia are common complaints. Balance problems and shoe wear difficulties are also issues. Soft tissue problems such as peroneal tendon tears and dislocation may also present. The patient can present with proximal/distal tibial stress fractures or fifth metatarsal zone II or III stress fractures. Medial ankle arthritis symptoms are seen in more advanced deformities with associated lateral instability. The physical exam should include observation of gait, range of motion, motor strength, and neurological exam. Hindfoot varus is best appreciated by the "peek-a-boo" sign (described by Manoli),[2] where one sees the medial heel when viewed from anteriorly. The high arch is best seen in the medial sagittal view. The Coleman block and Carroll tests can determine if the varus is forefoot driven (Figures 12-1 and 12-2). In the Coleman block test, the forefoot and hindfoot are placed on a 1-inch wood block with the first ray suspended off the block and the floor. If the hindfoot varus corrects, then this would represent forefoot-driven varus. However, if the hindfoot does not correct, then there is a hindfoot component as well (Figure 12-3). In the Carroll test, the patient is viewed from posterior off a step stool while the entire forefoot dangles over the edge. If the hindfoot varus corrects, then again the cavovarus is forefoot driven in a reciprocal manner. As is commonly seen in cavus feet, an equinus contracture should always be assessed. Gastrocnemius contracture should be accessed with the Silfverskiöld test. This is performed where the knee

Figure 12-1. Coleman and Carroll tests. (A) Coleman block test where the first ray is suspended of the wood block showing correction of hindfoot varus. (B) Carroll test with forefoot eliminated by suspending it over the step stool while the hind foot is in valgus.

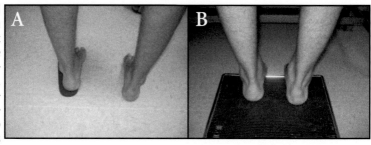

Figure 12-2. Observation. (A) Peek-a-boo sign of Manoli showing hindfoot varus when viewed from front. (B) Posterior view. (C, D) Coleman block test of left and right foot.

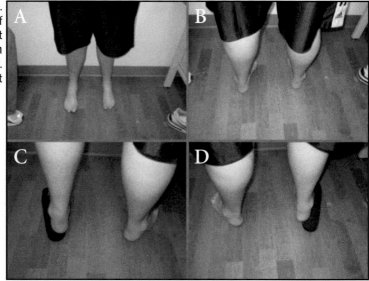

Figure 12-3. Charcot-Marie-Tooth I. (A) Frontal view of severe hindfoot varus. (B) Posterior view of hindfoot varus. (C) Coleman block test shows hindfoot does not correct when the first ray is eliminated. (D) Intrinsic weakness and atrophy with cross finger test.

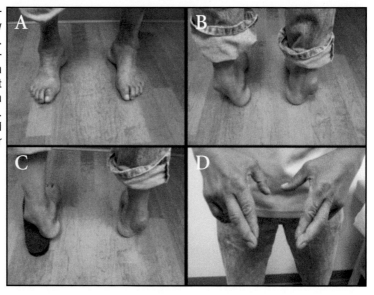

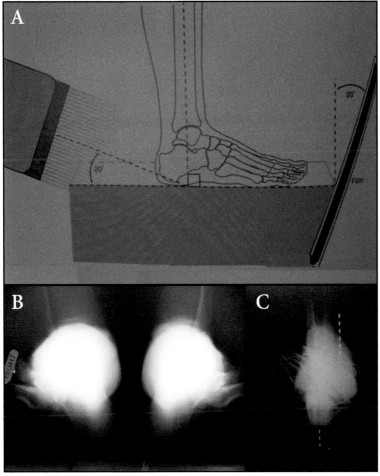

Figure 12-4. Hindfoot alignment view. (A) The x-ray beam is shot at a 20-degree angle in a posteroanterior orientation over a radiolucent stand. (B) Weight-bearing view depicting hindfoot varus. (C) Hindfoot alignment view with Coleman bock showing hindfoot correction when the first ray is eliminated.

is extended, the midfoot locked, and the ankle dorsiflexed. If the ankle does not come past neutral, then the gastrocnemius is considered tight. Furthermore, if the ankle still cannot come past neutral when flexing the knee, then the soleus or entire complex is considered involved. Radiographs should be weight bearing in the anteroposterior/lateral and hindfoot axial alignment views (Figure 12-4). The declination angle of Meary, calcaneal pitch, and hindfoot varus should be measured (Figure 12-4 B, C). A hindfoot alignment view with and without a Coleman block can also be performed. In vitro studies have shown increased medial ankle joint pressures with cavus of 10 degrees. Clinically, cavovarus can manifest with ankle instability, arthritis, as well as medial stress fractures of the distal tibia (Figure 12-5). Fractures of the lateral column of the foot involving the fourth or fifth metatarsals (zone II/III) may be seen (Figure 12-6). Peroneal tendon tears with or without retinacular instability are also common (Figure 12-7).

Figure 12-5. Ankle varus with arthritis. (A) Left ankle with medial arthritis and talar tilt. (B) Lateral view. (C) Hindfoot alignment view showing hindfoot varus. (D) Coleman block test with hindfoot alignment view without correction.

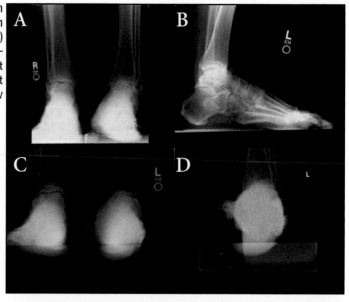

Figure 12-6. Zone III stress fracture driven varus. (A) Posteroanterior view. (B) Varus correction with Coleman block test. (C) Hindfoot alignment view. (D) Zone III stress fracture of the fifth metatarsal.

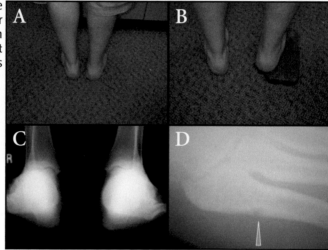

Figure 12-7. Peroneus longus II complex tear. (A) Proximal and distal tenodesis of peroneus longus to brevis. (B) Lateral foot X-ray. (C) Dorsally pre-bent 2-hole plate for fixation.

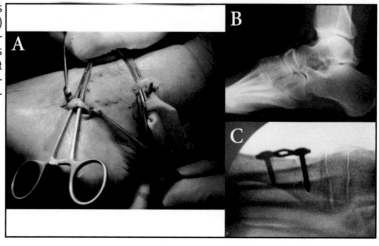

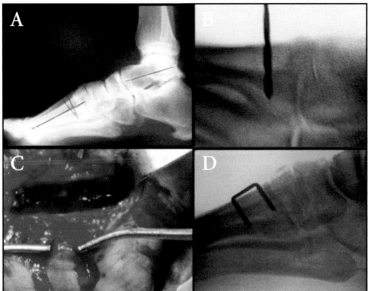

Figure 12-8. First metatarsal dorsal closing wedge basilar osteotomy. (A) Lateral radiograph with increased talar-first metatarsal declination angle. (B) Proximal predrilled fixation hole. (C) Four-mm dorsal wedge excision distal to pilot hole in B. (D) Fixation with staple.

Treatment

Given the previously indicated problems and the biomechanical problems with the locked foot, even asymptomatic patients may require treatment with simple methods, such as gastrocsoleus stretches and accommodative orthotic devices with first metatarsal head relief and lateral heel wedges. If any of the above conditions exist (eg, a peroneal tendon tear or zone II/III fracture of the fifth metatarsal), then reconstructive surgery also may be indicated and should be individualized. Depending on the exam and deficits, these may include tendon transfers and soft tissue releases and recessions. For anterior tibial tendon paralysis, a posterior tibial tendon transfer through the interosseous membrane can be done. A flexor hallucis longus transfer can be used for peroneal tendon paralysis. For an overactive peroneus longus, a tenotomy and side-to-side anastomosis with the brevis at a location below the lateral malleolus allowing a 1 to 2 cm lengthening will decrease its overdrive affect on the first metatarsal. For equinus contracture, the Strayer procedure will suffice. If the dorsiflexion is limited with the knee flexed, then a tendoachilles lengthening is indicated instead. Underlying structural problems should be stabilized. The pronated first ray can be corrected with a basilar dorsal closing wedge osteotomy for mild forefoot driven varus and first tarsometatarsal fusion with corrective osteotomy or lateral midtarsal closing wedge osteotomy for more severe deformities (see Figures 12-7 and 12-8). Osseous correction of the hindfoot with a Dwyer lateral closing wedge osteotomy is preferred over straight translation for hindfoot driven varus (Figure 12-9).[3] Once the foundation is corrected, the secondary pathology can be addressed, usually in the same setting. I will usually address the gastrocnemius complex first before performing all the necessary osseous procedures. Tendon transfers, ankle instability (eg, Broström), peroneal tendon repair with or without retinacular, and fibular groove reconstruction are performed at the end of the case.

Figure 12-9. Dwyer lateral closing wedge osteotomy. (A) Schanz 6-mm pin to aid reduction. (B) Two retrograde 7.3-mm cannulated cancellous lag screws.

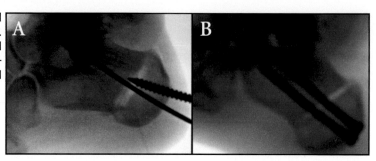

References

1. Guyton G. Current concepts review: orthopedic aspects of Charcot-Marie-Tooth disease. *Foot Ankle Int.* 2006;27(11):1003-1010.
2. Manoli A 2nd, Graham B. The subtle cavus foot, "the underpronator". *Foot Ankle Int.* 2005;26(3):256-263.
3. Kelikian AS. Calcaneal osteotomies. In: Kelikian AS, ed. *Operative Treatment of the Foot and Ankle.* Stamford, CT: Appleton & Lange; 1999:417-432.

I Am Performing a Triple Arthrodesis But Cannot Seem to Reduce the Talonavicular Joint. What Am I Doing Wrong?

Scott Nemec, DO and John G. Anderson, MD

When performing a triple arthrodesis, one needs to recognize the deformity that is being corrected. There are certainly times when the talonavicular joint does not seem to line up correctly. Recognizing the components that go into the deformity will assist in identifying roadblocks to overcome during correction, whether the procedure is being done for a flatfoot deformity or for a cavovarus deformity.

Most commonly, it is the flatfoot deformity that leads to frustration when trying to realign the talonavicular joint. The flatfoot deformity results from medial column incompetence, resulting in a forefoot varus and subsequent hindfoot valgus. This deformity invariably has an underlying equinus contracture. I believe the deformity is primarily driven by the equinus deformity, followed by forefoot varus as the medial column breaks down, and finally resulting in hindfoot valgus as the spring ligament and posterior tibial tendon fail. As a result of this, the forefoot and midfoot drift laterally into abduction, most commonly through the talonavicular joint with resulting dorsolateral peritalar subluxation (Figure 13-1). This manifests as talar uncoverage at the talonavicular joint. The hindfoot compensates and falls into valgus. A functionally short lateral column results and the talus plantarflexes as the calcaneus externally rotates (Figure 13-2).

Performing a triple arthrodesis is indicated when the flatfoot deformity becomes rigid, either as a result of degenerative changes in the subtalar, talonavicular, and calcaneocuboid articulations or through soft tissue contracture. This rigid deformity makes the joint-sparing procedures less attractive; therefore, triple arthrodesis is the treatment of choice. These deformities by nature tend to be stiffer than a typical flexible flatfoot, so appropriate soft tissue releases are needed to reposition the respective joints. This may include complete releases of the talonavicular, subtalar, and calcaneocuboid joints. The triple arthrodesis procedure should reverse the deformity at hand.

Figure 13-1. Anteroposterior view of foot demonstrates dorsolateral peritalar subluxation with talonavicular uncoverage. Also noted is the hallux valgus alignment of the first ray with uncoverage of the lateral sesamoid.

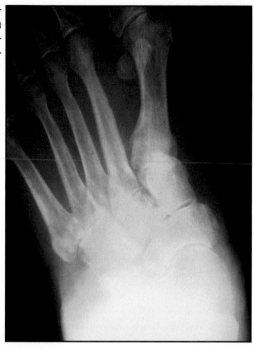

Figure 13-2. Lateral view of foot shows plantarflexed talus, ablation of the sinus tarsi, and collapse in midfoot.

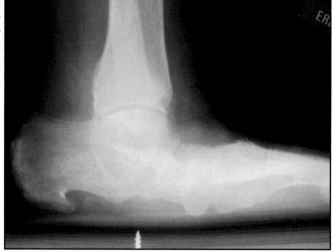

Accordingly, certain portions of the procedure may become difficult if the pathoanatomy of the foot is not understood. Typically, the deformity correction progresses from proximal to distal. Correcting the equinus deformity by standard tendoachilles lengthening or gastrocnemius recession helps reposition the hindfoot out of equinus and allows the talus and the calcaneus to dorsiflex. Preparing all joints for fusion ahead of time and performing appropriate capsular releases follow.

Initially, when performing a triple arthrodesis, the talus must be reduced on top of the calcaneus to its normal position on the posterior facet. In severe deformities, the calcaneus may actually sublux laterally in addition to tipping into valgus, so this must

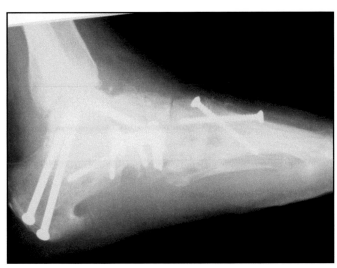

Figure 13-3. Lateral view of the foot after triple arthrodesis. Note restoration of the talus first metatarsal alignment, as well as talus location on calcaneus.

be addressed by medializing the calcaneus through the subtalar joint while derotating the subtalar joint at the same time. This is done by manually pushing the talus laterally while simultaneously pushing the calcaneus medially. Externally rotating the talus back onto the calcaneus and pushing it posteriorly will then bring the hindfoot out of valgus. This is performed by distraction longitudinally through the sinus tarsi using a laminar spreader between the lateral process of the talus and the anterior process of the calcaneus. When distraction occurs here, the talus externally rotates into its normal position relative to the calcaneus. Intraoperatively, you can appreciate the lateral process moving posteriorly relative to the angle of Gissane as the talus is pushed posteriorly and externally rotated. This can be challenging as this must be performed while maintaining manual correction of any lateral calcaneal subluxation. Having an assistant distract with the laminar spreader while I maintain medializing pressure on the calcaneus has been my most effective way of holding this until provisional fixation is achieved. Talar repositioning (dorsiflexion and external rotation) now moves the talus out of the way and allows the talonavicular joint to reduce by bringing the navicular medially and plantarly, thus correcting the dorsolateral peritalar subluxation (Figure 13-3). In essence, the midfoot abduction is thus corrected, and some of the forefoot varus (supination) is reduced around the talonavicular joint (Figure 13-4). There may sometimes be a gap in the talonavicular joint following this procedure. This should be anticipated, as the medial column needs to be shortened in order to correct the flatfoot deformity. Compressing this gap and obtaining bone-to-bone contact is necessary. This may require some adjustment in the amount of derotation performed as too much derotation will prevent compression of this space. Once bone-to-bone contact is established, this joint is stabilized first, followed by subtalar and calcaneocuboid joints. Fixation should only be implanted once adequate plantigrade alignment has been obtained. Provisional fixation may hold this position until definitive rigid fixation is applied. Medial column collapse coming from the talonavicular joint is now corrected, but residual forefoot supination must be corrected using additional distal medial column naviculocuneiform or tarsometatarsal fusions. When not performed correctly or completely, residual malalignment results.

Figure 13-4. Anteroposterior view foot after triple arthrodesis with medial column stabilization realignment at talonavicular articulation and correction of the associated hallux valgus deformity.

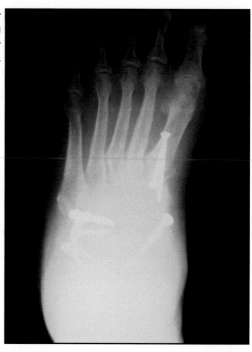

Suggested Readings

Hansen ST Jr, ed. *Functional Reconstruction of the Foot and Ankle*. Philadelphia, PA: Lippincott Williams and Wilkins; 2000.

Sammarco VJ, Magur EG, Sammarco GJ, Bagwe MR. Arthrodesis of the subtalar and talonavicular joints for correction of symptomatic hindfoot malalignment. *Foot Ankle Int*. 2006;27(9):661-666.

How Much Fixation Is Required for a Subtalar Fusion? What Is Your Postoperative Protocol?

Eric Breitbart, MD; Wayne Berberian, MD; and Sheldon Lin, MD

When performing a primary subtalar arthrodesis, you essentially have to decide between 1-screw and 2-screw fixation. To my knowledge, no hard Level I evidence exists in the literature to support or refute either technique. One must take into account the evidence available and make the best choice for the patient. While one screw may be enough for fixation in many cases, the risks and benefits of placement of a second screw should be considered. Complications of placing a second screw include additional operative time, increased risk of infection, as well as the potential for prominent hardware. However, when you compare those relatively minor risks, along with the biomechanical advantages of performing a 2-screw fixation versus the potential of not achieving adequate fixation of performing 1-screw fixation, I would always take the former. Therefore, in my personal practice, I always use double 4.5 mm or larger lag screws from the posteroinferior calcaneus to the anterior talar neck in a diverging orientation for fixation of primary subtalar fusions (Figure 14-1).

As I mentioned earlier, the literature is sparse regarding what is considered "adequate fixation" of a subtalar fusion. Chuckpaiwong et al, in a cadaver biomechanical study comparing fixation with a single talar neck screw, a single talar dome screw, double parallel screws, or double diverging screws, demonstrated that higher compressive force, torsional stiffness, and joint rotation resistance were achieved by double screw fixation compared to single screws.[1] Additionally, double diverging screws had higher torsional stiffness than double parallel screws, supporting my current practice.

In contrast, several retrospective studies (without a double screw group to compare results) have demonstrated successful fixation with only a single lag screw from the posteroinferior calcaneus to the anterior talar neck. In a 2004 study of 101 isolated subtalar arthrodesis, Haskel et al demonstrated a 98% success rate in fusion using a technique of single lag screw fixation from posteroinferior to anterosuperior across the posterior facet of the subtalar joint when combined with the application of an autograft taken from the floor of the sinus tarsi and anterior process.[2] Similarly, in a 2007 retrospective review of 92 subtalar arthrodesis with a single 7.0-mm partially threaded cancellous screw used

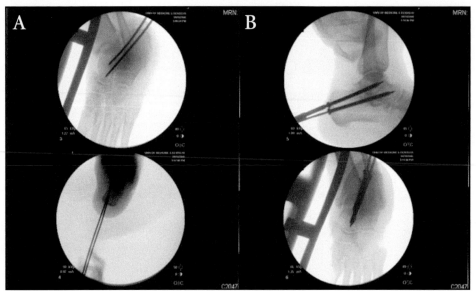

Figure 14-1. Intraoperative fluoroscopic images of subtalar arthrodesis using a double diverging screw technique. Note (A) the placement of the 2 guide wires from the posteroinferior calcaneus to the anterior talar neck followed by (B) fixation with 2 cannulated screws.

for fixation in addition to autogenous bone graft, Davies et al found that 95% of patients proceeded to undergo radiographic union and 93% achieved good or fair outcomes using the Angus and Cowell rating systems.[3] Furthermore, a study by Easley et al in 2000 demonstrated a union rate of 84% using single screw fixation versus 81% using double screw fixation.[4]

However, in spite of these data (which support a conclusion that fusion may be successfully achieved with single screw fixation), none of these studies provide the key answer as to what the long-term differences are between 1- and 2-screw fixations. My primary concern with the data on single screw subtalar fusion is that if adequate fixation is not achieved with that screw and the alignment even slightly shifts, poor biomechanical functionality may result, leading to the sequela of nonunion as well as arthritis in the surrounding joints and additional operations.

Finally, regarding the proper postoperative protocol for subtalar arthrodesis, it is important over the first 2 months to assure that no motion occurs at the subtalar joint and that no weight is borne by that joint. Optimally, this is achieved by placing a compliant patient in a short leg cast. Following this initial period of nonweight bearing (minimum 8 weeks), the patient should slowly progress to full weight bearing in the cast as to not overstress the fusion site. This principle should be followed not just for subtalar arthrodesis, but for all fusion procedures that you perform. My specific postoperative protocol following a subtalar fusion is to maintain the patient nonweight bearing in a short leg cast for the first 8 weeks postsurgery. Over the course of the next month, I slowly progress the patient from 20% of full weight bearing to full weight bearing while still in the cast or Controlled Ankle Movement walker. Once the patient is fully weight bearing, I would remove the cast and start the patient on a course of physical therapy 3 times per week for an additional 6 weeks in order to assist the patient in regaining functionality in the remainder of the ankle. My regular follow-up for these patients includes visits at 1, 2, and 4 weeks, followed by monthly visits until radiographic union has been achieved. I assess my patients radiographically beginning at 2 weeks postoperatively and every 4 weeks until successful union has occurred.

References

1. Chuckpaiwong B, Easley ME, Glisson RR. Screw placement in subtalar arthrodesis: a biomechanical study. *Foot Ankle Int.* 2009;30(2):133-141.
2. Haskell A, Pfeiff C, Mann R. Subtalar joint arthrodesis using a single lag screw. *Foot Ankle Int.* 2004;25(11):774-777.
3. Davies MB, Rosenfeld PF, Stavrou P, Saxby TS. A comprehensive review of subtalar arthrodesis. *Foot Ankle Int.* 2007;28(3):295-297.
4. Easley ME, Trnka HJ, Schon LC, Myerson MS. Isolated subtalar arthrodesis. *J Bone Joint Surg Am.* 2000;82(5):613-624.

SECTION III

ANKLE

How Do I Treat a Patient With Recurrent Medial Ankle Pain and a Magnetic Resonance Imaging Finding of Medial Malleolar Edema Consistent With a Medial Malleolar Stress Fracture?

David R. Richardson, MD

Because of the increased stress placed on the medial aspect of the ankle and the vertical orientation often associated with a medial malleolar stress fracture, treatment of this condition can be frustrating for both the physician and the patient. Although the pathogenesis is not clear, the vertical appearance of the fracture line is similar to that seen in supination-adduction ankle fractures.[1-3] Ankle dorsiflexion and internal rotation of the talus may cause repetitive stress on the medial malleolus. Patients with excessive foot pronation, tibia vara, or genu varum (bowed legs at or below the knee) may be more prone to this injury.[4] Those with a cavovarus foot posture may also be at risk as well. Limited transverse tarsal motion in this population increases stress across the ankle, which may cause a vertical stress fracture of the medial malleolus.[1-4]

Treatment of any patient begins with a thorough history and physical. The typical patient with a medial malleolar stress fracture is an athlete in his second or third decade participating in repetitive running and jumping activities. Carefully investigate for possible menstrual irregularities, hormonal imbalances, nutritional deficiencies, and metabolic disorders.[5] Be especially careful in the evaluation of competitive female athletes as many will have associated disorders. Ask the patient about any changes in his or her workout or diet. Is the pain constant or activity related? Do certain activities or lower extremity positions exacerbate the pain? Most patients complain of vague medial ankle pain without a history of instability. On physical exam, carefully evaluate the ankle range of motion and stability. Usually there are no significant findings in this regard. There will be tenderness with palpation over the medial malleolus and often with dorsiflexion and internal rotation of the talus in the ankle mortis. There may be a palpable anterior medial spur as well.[6]

Figure 15-1. MRI shows medial malleolar stress fracture before it is visible on plain radiographs.

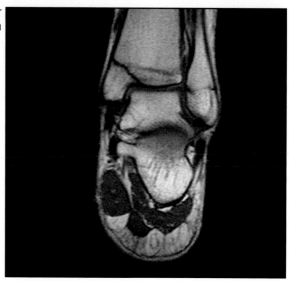

The differential diagnosis includes tibial periostitis (shin splints), posterior tibial tendonitis, deltoid or spring ligament strain, medial malleolar avulsion fractures, medial osteochondral lesions, and nerve entrapment. Usually you can localize the pain over the medial malleolus rather than the more inferiorly located deltoid or posteriorly located posterior tibial tendon.

You must always obtain standing ankle radiographs that include lateral, anteroposterior, and mortise views, although these often are negative for up to 2 months.[1-3,7] A bone scan or magnetic resonance imaging (Figure 15-1) is more sensitive than radiographs for confirming a stress fracture, but it is often difficult to determine whether the fracture line is complete or incomplete. I often obtain a computed tomography (CT) scan to guide treatment. A CT scan possesses the resolution needed to assess both orientation and extent of the fracture. It also is helpful preoperatively to plan for appropriate hardware and the possible need for bone graft. In addition, anterior medial spurs or osteochondral lesions may be better evaluated.

Treatment is based on several factors. The chronicity of symptoms, timing of the athlete's season, and athletic level all must be considered. It is important that the patient and physician are clear about expectations as this may guide treatment as well. Nonoperative treatment may take up to 2 months longer to fully heal versus operative treatment.[1-4,7] Also, it is important to determine if the fracture line is complete or incomplete.

My preference is to treat a young patient with an acute, incomplete fracture with immobilization and nonweight bearing for 4 weeks. You can then progress weight bearing over the next 4 weeks. Full activity can begin in a functional brace at that time. In an older patient with a medial malleolar stress fracture, a more structural brace (eg, Arizona brace [ArizonaAFO, Mesa, AZ]) is often warranted. These patients often overload the medial aspect of their ankles because of increased valgus ankle forces (usually a result of posterior tibial insufficiency and/or deltoid incompetence). I often place these patients in a weight-bearing cast for 8 weeks while the brace is being fabricated. I ask patients to wear the brace for about 1 year, then I can often transition them into custom orthotics with good medial support.

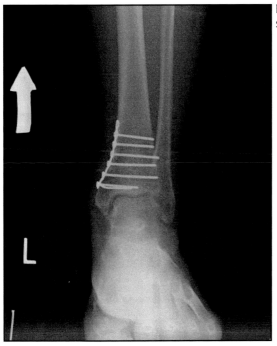

Figure 15-2. Fixation of medial malleolar stress fracture with buttress plate and screws.

Patients with complete fractures on x-ray or CT, especially with any displacement, will need surgery. If the fracture is vertically oriented, consider a buttress plate (Figure 15-2), although 2 screws placed perpendicular to the fracture are acceptable as well. This may be performed in a percutaneous manner if nondisplaced. If there is a nonunion or any displacement, consider an open approach with bone grafting of the fracture site. Bone spurs and soft-tissue impingement lesions must be removed as well. Postoperatively, patients need to be nonweight bearing for 8 weeks or until radiographic healing has occurred. I take the cast off at 4 weeks after surgery and begin range-of-motion exercises either in physical therapy or at home, depending on patient reliability and activity level. I place patients in a custom orthosis with a ¼-inch heel lift for 1 year post injury. I believe this protects against both valgus and dorsiflexion stress.

I now place all patients with a stress fracture on calcium and vitamin D_3 supplementation if there are no contraindications. Vitamin D_3 has a very high therapeutic index and toxicity is rare. Patients are told to be sensitive to worsening symptoms and may simply limit their activity for a few days at the first sign of pain. This usually prevents recurrence if predisposing factors were treated initially.

References

1. Orava S, Karpakka J, Taimela S, et al. Stress fracture of the medial malleolus. *J Bone Joint Surg Am*. 1995;77:362-365.
2. Shabat S, Sampson KB, Mann G, et al. Stress fractures of the medial malleolus—a review of the literature and report of a 15-year-old elite gymnast. *Foot Ankle Int*. 2002;23:647-650.
3. Shelbourne KD, Fisher DA, Rettig AC, McCarroll JR. Stress fractures of the medial malleolus. *Am J Sports Med*. 1988;16:60-63.

4. Brockwell J, Yeung Y, Griffith JF. Stress fractures of the foot and ankle. *Sports Med Arthrosc.* 2009;17:149-159.
5. Lappe J, Cullen D, Haynatzki G, et al. Calcium and vitamin D supplementation decreases incidence of stress fracture in female navy recruits. *J Bone Miner Res.* 2008;23:741-749.
6. Jowett AJ, Birks CL, Blackney MC. Medial malleolar stress fractures secondary to chronic ankle impingement. *Foot Ankle Int.* 2008;29:716-721.
7. Boden BP, Osbahr DC. High-risk stress fractures: evaluation and treatment. *J Am Acad Orthop Surg.* 2000;8:344-353.

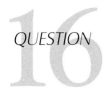

WHICH OSTEOCHONDRAL TALAR LESIONS NEED SURGERY?

Christopher Bibbo, DO, FACS, FAAOS

Osteochondral lesions of the talus (OLT) are a very common finding after injury, typically including sprains and ankle fractures. It is generally accepted that OLT occur in up to 15% of severe sprains and ankle fractures. In addition to acute traumatic OLT, OLT also include those generated from repetitive micro trauma, such as chronic lateral ankle instability as well as idiopathic causes and medications such as steroids (eg, osteochondritis dissecans). The question of whether to perform operative intervention in these patients demands the surgeon to evaluate the clinical situation on several levels. There are several classification systems for OLT based on plain radiographs (Bernt & Hardy classification[1]), computed tomography (CT) scan, and magnetic resonance imaging (MRI classification[2]). All have their particular utility based on assessment needs. All OLT classification systems are somewhat arbitrary, and thus the author prefers not to quantitate necessity of treatment based solely on imaging classifications. Imaging studies are only one piece of the puzzle when evaluating OLT, and patient history and symptomatology must be assessed.

The setting of the patient history and clinical presentation are very important. The first setting to be considered is the presentation of the acute OLT. Acutely diagnosed talar OLT may be observed provided that the lesions do not involve a large bony portion of the talus or are not significantly displaced (2+ mm). Displaced osteochondral lesions that are traumatic in nature need to be reduced and fixed in the acute setting. My preference, if the lesion is large enough, is acute fixation. Outside of this setting, osteochondral lesions of 1 cm or less can generally be observed and treated in the acute setting with nonweight bearing and limited mobilization of the ankle. This can be done for several weeks in order to allow an adequate reparative process to occur. In the subacute setting (greater than 6 to 8 weeks), presentation of a patient with a new diagnosis of an OLT or a patient with a known diagnosis that has been inadequately treated warrants an additional trial of conservative treatment, including nonweight bearing, limited mobilization, followed by full range of motion and weight bearing based on the progression of x-rays. If x-rays fail to show a reparative process that is adequate, the surgeon is often required to perform a further investigation including that of MRI and CT. Because plain radiographs are only

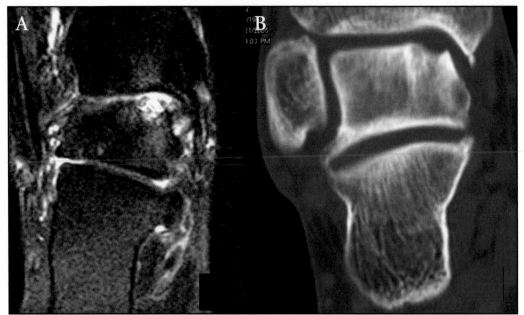

Figure 16-1. (A) T2 MRI and (B) CT of chronic talar OLT. Note the vastly improved bone detail on CT in subacute lesions.

a threshold study for OLT and do not provide the wealth of information often desired in evaluating the talar OLT, further imaging is warranted. High-resolution MRI used to image OLT will universally reveal surrounding bone edema. The condition of the overlying cartilage may be further assessed with an arthrogram performed in conjunction with the MRI. However, the distinct disadvantage of an MRI is that MRIs tend to "over-read" lesions in both the acute and chronic settings. In the acute setting, bone marrow edema may mask bone detail; bone edema may last for up to 6 months after an acute traumatic injury, obscuring fine bone changes. In the chronic setting, repetitive micro trauma can also induce additional bone edema. Thus, in the author's opinion, the overly sensitive MRI can over-read the area of injury and does not give a good picture of the fine architectural details of the bone. Typically, the author prefers an MRI at 1 to 3 months; thereafter, a CT is preferred to evaluate OLT. Thus, the author's goal for evaluating all subacute OLT is to evaluate the bone quality. CT provides superior detail on the bony architecture and may be used alone or in conjunction with early MRI findings. Thus, the author's preferred imaging modality for all subacute talar OLT is a CT scan (Figure 16-1). A special note should be made to incidental lesions found on imaging exams that are otherwise asymptomatic. There are no data to support surgically pursuing "incidentaloma OLT" that are asymptomatic. However, larger OLT discovered in such a manner should be followed at least yearly. Additionally, because many OLT will change over time,[3] reimaging may also be indicated. The author consistently uses the above-stated imaging modalities within the stated time frames for reimaging OLT.

A special note is the occurrence of OLT in skeletally immature individuals. In this setting, a more generous period of conservative management is warranted, as it is believed (hoped) the reparative potential in the skeletally immature patient is greater than that of adults. However, careful scrutiny must be made of imaging studies, especially in large

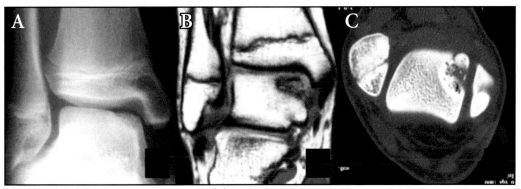

Figure 16-2. (A) Plain radiograph and (B) MRI of an unusually large talar OLT in a 15-year-old male. (C) CT clearly demonstrates poor bone quality of the OLT bed. Although youth typically allows more valiant attempts at conservative treatment, lesions of this quality/size indicate poor healing potential that will ultimately require operative management. The physis may be spared by careful planning of osteotomies. Long-term patient follow-up is required.

OLT in adolescents because large lesions with poor bone features herald a guarded prognosis, even in skeletally immature patients (Figure 16-2).

In those patients who are entering the chronic phase (greater than 3 months), CT scan is warranted to evaluate the fine bony architecture. During the transition from the subacute into the chronic setting, the evaluation of the bony architecture of OLT is especially important because, at this point, persistent pain is not just a cartilaginous problem. A large component of the pain is due to the poor reparative process of the bone. Thus, the goal of surgical intervention, when indicated, is to provide a source of cartilage and bone for a reparative process. It does the surgeon no good to concentrate solely on restoring the cartilage surface when the bone is involved and untreated. For these reasons, the author prefers to obtain CTs on all patients who are in the transition from the subacute into the chronic phase.

The first item in the workup must assess the acuity of the injury and progression of the reparative process of both bone and cartilage. The next issue to address is the size of the OLT. In general, I try to semiquantify the size (mm, cm); a common (empiric) gauge for OLT is less than 10 mm or greater than 10 mm. The next item to assess is the location of the OLT. Although the medial OLT have been the most common in the author's practice, there are a large number of lesions that occur on the lateral dome of the talus. MRI data have demonstrated that 62% of OLT (which tend to be larger) reside within the medial dome, while the lateral dome houses 34% of talar OLT. The mid-equator of the talus is the most common location on both medial and lateral shoulders of the talus; the central portion of the talus is much less affected by OLT.[4] The plafond must also be assessed for osteochondral lesions, with plafond osteochondral lesions occurring with an OLT in up to 16% of patients.[5] Although fanciful, exact "kissing" lesions of the talar dome/tibial plafond are uncommon.[5]

The most important task in evaluating OLT is the integration of the patient's clinical history and physical examination with the imaging studies. This portion of the clinical assessment must also include a thorough examination of the ankle, including tenderness, range of motion, associated global ankle issues such as ankle ligament instability, peroneal tendon pathology, neuromuscular disease, foot type (cavus, pes planus), bony

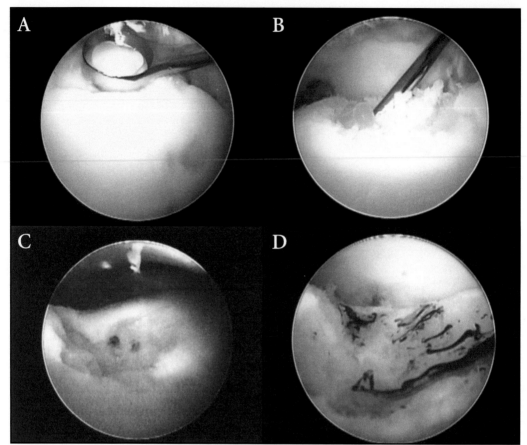

Figure 16-3. Arthroscopic débridement and microdrilling of talar OLT. (A) Curettage of lesion back to a stable rim, followed by (B, C) drilling. (D) Release of pump flow confirms adequate depth of drilling to viable, bleeding bone. These efforts will assist with recruitment of osteochondral precursor cells and the development of stable fibrocartilage cap.

deformity (eg, distal tibial varus), and functional demands (athletics, work, etc). It is imperative to stratify patients into "untreated" and "previously treated" categories, assessing what treatments have failed and why, and how to avoid the same pitfalls. All treatments and success or set-backs must be determined. It must be ascertained if the patient is still symptomatic and if the patient is functional. It is the author's opinion that nonoperative treatment is indicated first in patients in the acute setting who have been referred and treatment has not been done. We attempt to do this for 2 to 3 months. If there is continued pain and lack of progressive healing and further investigations provide evidence that the reparative process is not progressing along as well as we would like to see within that time frame (via imaging studies), the next determination is which type of surgical intervention is warranted.

The surgical interventions that are warranted in the acute phase include microdrilling or microfracturing techniques (Figure 16-3), osteochondral transplant techniques (Figure 16-4), as well as autologous chondrocyte implantation techniques. In the author's experience, microdrilling and microfracture appear to perform best in lesions less than 8 mm and in acute lesions that are treated early. It is also this author's experience that OLT that

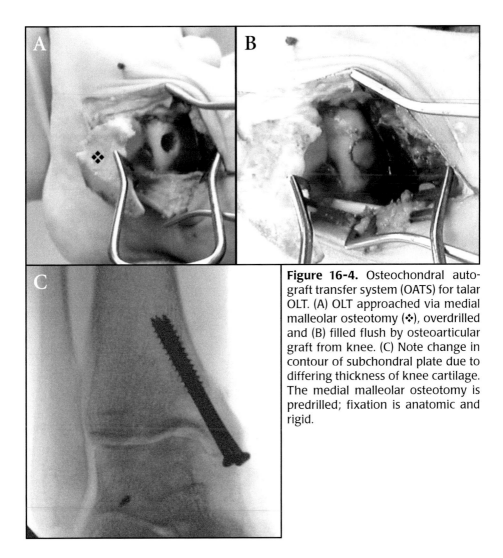

Figure 16-4. Osteochondral autograft transfer system (OATS) for talar OLT. (A) OLT approached via medial malleolar osteotomy (❖), overdrilled and (B) filled flush by osteoarticular graft from knee. (C) Note change in contour of subchondral plate due to differing thickness of knee cartilage. The medial malleolar osteotomy is predrilled; fixation is anatomic and rigid.

have been untreated (including conservative measures) for longer than 4 to 6 months regardless of size, and definitely those larger than 1 cm, respond poorly to microdrilling and microfracture techniques. Therefore, this author relegates microdrilling and microfracture techniques solely to those lesions that are less than 1 cm in size and are being treated early in the acute phase and those OLT that are in the transition phase from the acute to the subacute period. Microfracture and microdrilling can be done by a number of techniques, but arthroscopic techniques are preferred over open techniques and can be easily performed by using 30- and 70-degree arthroscopy equipment and microvector drill guides. The author prefers to use a 0.62-pointed Kirschner wire or a pointed bone reduction tool such as a dental pick to obtain good microfracture footprints to a depth of 3 mm below the subchondral plate (see Figure 16-3). After drilling and microfracturing, the author will allow immediate mobility of the ankle based on the wound but will limit the weight bearing for 4 weeks for lesions less than 1 cm, and 4 to 8 weeks for lesions greater than 1 cm. For lesions that are greater than 1 cm, especially those that are past the subacute phase and into the chronic phase, the author has found that the great majority of these lesions tend to fail microdrilling techniques. Therefore, the author prefers to go directly to an osteochondral autograft transfer system (OATS; Arthrex, Inc, Naples, FL) procedure (see Figure 16-4). The OATS can harvest and allow the utilization of native tissues, as well as allograft tissues. Anatomic areas that are suggested suitable for harvest to treat OLT include the knee, the calcaneocuboid joint, the undersurface of the navicular, and the anterior portion of the lateral talar facet. However, the author finds that the best geometric match is usually obtained from talar allografts (fresh or frozen) or from the knee. When taken from the knee, the author prefers not to take the graft arthroscopically, but rather through a mini-open procedure, which allows exact identification and study of the contour of the cartilage to match the talar defect. Knee range of motion is performed as soon as the wound allows, within the first 7 days postoperatively. Quad sets are begun immediately. The donor site area is generally back filled with demineralized bone matrix (DBM) material or a tricalcium phosphate material, both of which appear to decrease bone pain.

Allografts are a well known source for osteoarticular material. The fresh allografts are generally regarded as having a large number of live cells that regenerate; however, frozen allografts seem to have adequate results. The author reserves the use of fresh allografts for large defects such as areas that require greater than 20% to 25% of the mediolateral talar dome, where a particular contour must be followed. Using any type of OATS system, this surgeon prefers to treat an area by this technique when only 2 plugs are needed. When getting into a situation where 3 or more plugs are needed, the surgeon should consider the use of a talar allograft to get an exact match of that area. Utilization of these talar allografts generally requires an osteotomy, which can be a simple oblique osteotomy or a chevron, but it should be noted that all osteotomies should be predrilled and finished with a fine osteotome. Adequate exposure is obtained by releasing the anteroposterior ankle joint capsule and part of the posterior fibro-osseous tendon bed and ligaments. The posterior tibial tendon must be protected at all times. After obtaining an adequate size and fit, the patient is allowed early range of motion based on the behavior of the surgical incision. Weight bearing is reserved until there is radiographic evidence of healing of the medial malleolus, at which time toe-touch weight-bearing is begun. Generally, full weight bearing is not begun for 8 to 10 weeks postoperatively. Tips for obtaining an adequate and proper fitting large talar allograft include the following[6,7]:

- Hold the allograft in femoral head holder (vice) while carving out the match.
- Use imprint transfer techniques: Mark the edges of the defect with a marking pen, transfer to a glove wrapper, and then transfer this to the graft surface overlying the template to match the defect in order to obtain an exact configuration that matches the OLT (or, use sterile foil from suture package).
- Take care to harvest the graft material: A graft should be taken slightly larger and trimmed down gradually to fit.
- Grafts should never be prominent, but rather flush: Slightly subsided is more acceptable than proud.
- Use an impaction device that overhangs the graft to help prevent an excessively subsided fit.
- Be as gentle as possible as even mild cycles of impaction have a negative impact on cartilage health.

One must be aware that when a graft is taken from the talus, radiographs will demonstrate a match in the height of the subchondral plate. However, when grafts are taken from the knee, radiographs will reveal a subchondral plate that is lower in position due to the increased thickness of the knee cartilage (see Figure 16-4).

The use of retrograde drilling has been popularized by Taranow and co-workers.[8] In this technique, ankle arthroscopy is employed to place a drill vector guide directed through the sinus tarsi, with the drill path opening onto the talar OLT. After retrograde drilling of the OLT, the drill path and OLT cavity are back filled with graft material. This technique may be useful for the so-called "cystic blow-out" lesion (OLT with an "intact" cartilage cap), but pose the difficulty of assessing the correct placement of the guide intra-operatively. Unless a large voided cystic area is present and readily visible on fluoroscopy and arthroscopy, the lesion may be missed because of the intact cartilage cap. Taranow et al have recommended the direct instillation of contrast dye to ascertain complete packing of the drill tunnel and cystic lesion. Taranow et al's technique is best relegated to isolated medial shoulder lesions. Large volume cystic lesions may be successfully treated with bulk fresh osteoarticular allografts.[9] Multi-cystic areas with tunnels are best managed via an open talar procedure. All cystic cavities and tunnels should be drilled prior to filling to allow vascular ingrowth into the area. The author recommends autologous bone, which may be supplemented with DBM if need be, thereby extending the graft.

A special comment should be made regarding the use of synthetic and xenograft materials in the treatment of talar OLT. Recently, "porous" products composed of poly(lactide-co-glycolide)/polyglycolide, "crystalline copolymers," polylactide with calcium sulfate, and photo-oxidized bovine bone have been promoted as suitable substitutes for bone in managing talar OLT and for back filling OATS harvest sites. However, reports from both the knee literature[10] and the foot-ankle literature[11] clearly do not support the use of such products. The author's experience with these products also does not lend support to their use in the management of talar OLT (or any other bone void issue). The only treatment, in this surgeon's opinion, for OLT that involves cartilage or cartilage plus bone is exact replacement: cartilage or cartilage plus bone. The author's rank order for tissue grafting materials for talar OLT is as follows: autograft tissue, fresh allograft, frozen allograft, freeze-dried allograft. Demineralized bone powder, bone morphogenetic protein-2, and platelet-rich plasma are acceptable adjuvants to assist with the bone phase healing.[12] Thus, at the time of this writing, any other materials used as the primary modality for the treatment of talar OLT are unproven and considered unacceptable.

Conclusion

OLT most commonly occur on the medial dome of the talus and are to be suspected after persistent ankle pain lasting greater than 8 to 10 weeks after an ankle injury. Pain is typically deep and worse with weight bearing and direct palpation in plantarflexion. Conservative measure such as restricted weight bearing and immobilization are warranted in the acute phase. Surgical intervention is indicated in properly selected patients with a corroborating history and physical examination and concordant imaging results. MRI is valuable in the early phase (less 12 weeks) to assess early OLT. Because subacute OLT indicate not only a cartilage issue but also a persistent bone healing issue, beyond

12 weeks, CT adds greater detail to the underlying bony architecture. Clinical situations that generally require surgical intervention include the following:

- OLT with large bony components that are displaced
- Smaller OLT that have failed appropriate conservative treatments
- Painful OLT that have been untreated/undertreated and present beyond 3 months from the index event
- Progression of an OLT with concordant symptomatology
- OLT that have been previously treated with a microfracture technique that have failed or recurred, or those that have been treated by other techniques with failure of that technique with persistent pain

References

1. Berndt AL, Harty M. Transchondral fractures (osteochondritis dissecans) of the talus. *J Bone Joint Surg Am.* 1959;41:988-1020.
2. Hepple S, Winson IG, Glew D. Osteochondral lesions of the talus: a revised classification. *Foot Ankle Int.* 1999;20(12):789-793.
3. Elias I, Jung JW, Raikin SM, Schweitzer MW, Carrio JA, Morrison WB. Osteochondral lesions of the talus: change in MRI findings over time in talar lesions without operative intervention and implications for staging systems. *Foot Ankle Int.* 2006;27(3):157-166.
4. Elias I, Zoga AC, Morrison WB, Besser M, Schweitzer ME, Rainin SM. Osteochondral lesions of the talus: localization and morphologic data from 424 patients using a novel anatomical grid scheme. *Foot Ankle Int.* 2007;28(2):154-161.
5. Elias I, Raikin S, Schweitzer ME, Besser MP, Morrison WB, Zoga AC. Osteochondral lesions of the distal tibial plafond: localization and morphologic characteristics with an anatomical grid. *Foot Ankle Int.* 2009;30(6):524-529.
6. Chen CT, Burton-Wurster N, Borden C, Hueffer K, Bloom SE, Lust G. Chondrocyte necrosis and apoptosis in impact damaged articular cartilage. *J Orthop Res.* 2001;19(4):703-711.
7. Milentijevic D, Rubel IF, Liew AS, Helfet DL, Torzilli PA. An in vivo rabbit model for cartilage trauma: a preliminary study of the influence of impact stress magnitude on chondrocyte death and matrix damage. *J Orthop Trauma.* 2005;19(7):466-473.
8. Taranow WS, Bisignani GA, Towers JD, Conti SF. Retrograde drilling of osteochondral lesions of the medial talar dome. *Foot Ankle Int.* 1999;20(8):474-480.
9. Raikin SM. Fresh osteochondral allografts for large-volume cystic osteochondral defects of the talus. *J Bone Joint Surg Am.* 2009;91(12):2818-2826.
10. Adams MR, Gehrmann RM, Bibbo C, Garcia JP, Najarian RG, Patel DV. In vivo assessment of incorporation of bone graft substitute plugs in osteoarticular autograft transplant surgery. Paper presented at: American Orthopaedic Society for Sports Medicine Annual Meeting Final Program; July 15-18, 2010; Providence, RI.
11. Lin JS, Andersen LB, Juliano PJ. Effectiveness of composite bone graft substitute plugs in the treatment of chondral and osteochondral lesions of the talus. *J Foot Ankle Surg.* 2010;49(3):224-232.
12. Bibbo C, Hatfield PS. Platelet-rich plasma concentrate to augment bone fusion. *Foot Ankle Clin.* 2010;15(4):641-649.

WHEN DO YOU PERFORM AN ALLOGRAFT OR AUTOGRAFT TALAR TRANSPLANTATION GRAFT FOR A FAILED OSTEOCHONDRAL TALAR LESION?

Gregory C. Berlet, MD and Jaymes D. Granata, MD

Osteochondral lesions of the talus (OLT) represent a wide spectrum of cartilage and subchondral bone defects of the talar dome. The etiology is multifactorial, divided into primary and secondary causes. Primary lesions are related to intrinsic host factors, including chronic disease and genetic predisposition. The exact mechanisms of primary OLT are not completely understood, but the common endpoint is likely a deficient blood supply to the subchondral bone. Secondary OLT are the result of mechanical stress, including malalignment, instability, and trauma. There are 2 common patterns of OLT. Anterolateral lesions are almost exclusively associated with an acute traumatic event, where ankle dorsiflexion and inversion cause the anterolateral portion of the talus to impinge on the fibula. Posteromedial lesions are more often associated with both primary and secondary causes.

Our treatment recommendations depend on patient demographics and the stage of the lesion. Staging OLT can be done with a variety of different imaging studies. We begin our evaluation with standard weight-bearing radiographs of the ankle (Figure 17-1). To better understand the location and extent of a lesion noted on x-ray, we often utilize magnetic resonance imaging (MRI) scans, especially for preoperative planning. Most recent classification systems for OLT are based on the classic staging system proposed by Berndt and Harty.[1] Subsequent authors have modified this original staging system to reflect the interpretations of advanced imaging techniques. An MRI-based staging system by Hepple et al[2] classifies lesions as 1 through 5:

1. Stage 1 lesions are isolated cartilage defects.

2. Stage 2A lesions are cartilage lesions with underlying subchondral bone fracture and edema.

3. Stage 2B lesions are stage 2A lesions without edema.

4. Stage 3 lesions are detached lesions that are not displaced.

Figure 17-1. Antero-posterior and mortise views demonstrating a medial talar dome lesion.

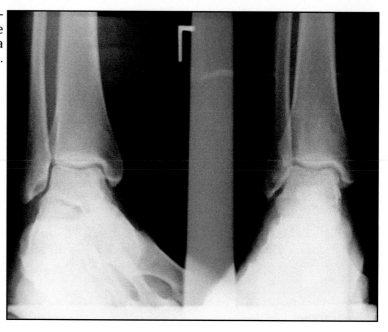

5. Stage 4 lesions are displaced.

6. Stage 5 lesions have subchondral cyst formation.[2]

Despite the numerous classification systems, no one system appears to be ideal with regard to prognosis and treatment recommendations. Even advanced staged lesions may respond favorably to conservative management. With this in mind, our initial treatment protocol includes conservative management in the majority of cases. The exception to this rule is an acute injury with a displaced fragment that would be amenable to internal fixation. Otherwise, a trial of immobilization and rest followed by physical therapy over a 6-week period may significantly decrease the patient's symptoms. If conservative management is prolonged despite persisting symptoms, the outcome of any future surgical procedure may become compromised. Waiting longer than 1 year to perform surgery has been found to result in inferior outcomes compared to more prompt surgical interventions.[3] We will discuss the different surgical options available to our patients who remain symptomatic after 6 weeks of conservative management.

Our surgical recommendations vary based on the patient's age, activity level, expectations, and associated pathology, such as tibiotalar arthritis. Lesion-specific variables include the size and location of the OLT and the duration of symptoms. With this information, surgical options can be divided into 3 major categories[4]:

1. Retaining the fragment and securing it in place with internal fixation, or drilling and bone grafting procedures.

2. Removing the fragment and stimulating fibrocartilage formation through débridement and microfracture.

3. Removing the fragment and transplanting hyaline cartilage to the defect. This can be achieved with either autograft or allograft transplantation.

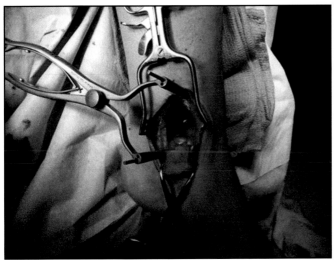

Figure 17-2. Exposure of the medial talar dome. A predrilled chevron medial malleolar osteotomy is reflected distally. Distraction is achieved with pins in the talus and tibia using a Hintermann distractor (Integra LifeSciences Corporation, Plainsboro, NJ).

For patients who have either failed conservative management or failed an initial surgical procedure for OLT, we will consider cartilage transplantation procedures in certain circumstances. We reserve bulk allograft transplantation for patients with large (>3 cm^2) unconfined shoulder lesions of the talar dome where the anatomy would not be appropriately restored with autograft osteochondral plugs. We use only fresh allograft transplants to optimize the chondrocyte viability after surgery. Patients who are candidates for this procedure are placed on a transplant list. Once a donor is identified, the patient is notified and surgery in performed within 48 hours.

In smaller, contained lesions, we use either osteochondral autografts or allograft, depending on patient characteristics such as weight and activity level. For autograft procedures, we use the osteochondral autograft transfer system (OATS; Arthrex, Inc, Naples, FL) to harvest cartilage from the ipsilateral knee. Depending on the location of the lesion, a medial malleolar osteotomy may be necessary to adequately expose the defect and perform the transplantation (Figure 17-2). We prefer to use one larger plug as opposed to multiple smaller plugs (mosaicplasty) for the majority of our cases. The plug is inserted perpendicular to the surface and flush with the apex of the surrounding cartilage (Figure 17-3). The predrilled chevron osteotomy is secured with 2 partially threaded cancellous screws (Figure 17-4).

Patients must be aware of the potential donor site morbidity associated with this autograft procedure. The ideal patient for autograft transplantation has no history of ipsilateral knee pain or trauma and is not overweight. Obesity may be considered a relative contraindication due to a higher incidence of poor outcomes related to the donor site.[5] Due to the possible complications with autograft, we have shifted toward using fresher allograft matched for size and side.

There are still many unanswered questions regarding the management of OLT. We are continually reviewing our patient data to better understand the outcomes of our treatment. We are particularly interested in refining surgical indications and understanding the association between certain variables and prognosis, including patient age, size of the lesion, and bone marrow edema.

Figure 17-3. Osteochondral auto-graft transplantation. The plug is inserted flush with the highest point of the medial talar dome.

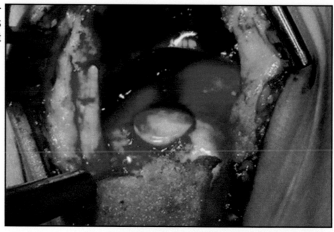

Figure 17-4. Restoration of the medial talar dome contour with the autogenous autograft plug. Medial malleolar osteotomy fixation with 2 partially threaded cancellous screws.

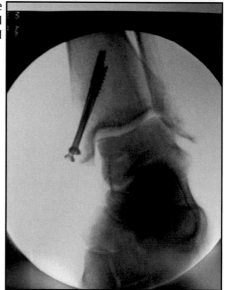

We have found that size does matter when it comes to OLT, with larger lesions more often requiring surgery to relieve the patient's symptoms. Lesions over 1 cm² have inconsistent results with microfracture, and a transplantation procedure may be the initial procedure of choice for some of these smaller lesions.

Patient age also appears to be directly related to surgical outcomes, with younger patients generally reporting better overall results. Historically, patients with open growth plates were associated with the best healing potential. We have found that patients younger than 20 years old have increased healing potential, independent of growth plate activity.

Bone marrow edema can be helpful in defining the prognosis after an initial surgical intervention with microfracture. We consider the presence of persistent bone marrow edema on MRI at 1 year to be a strong indication that microfracture is failing.

Collectively, we hope that these data will better define the surgical indications and surgical procedures of choice in OLT, eliminating the potential morbidity associated with failed conservative management and repeat surgical procedures.

References

1. Berndt AL, Harty M. Transchondral fractures (osteochondritis dissecans) of the talus. *J Bone Joint Surg.* 1959;41A:988-1020.
2. Hepple S, Winson IG, Glew D. Osteochondral lesions of the talus: a revised classification. *Foot Ankle Int.* 1999;20(12):789-793.
3. Pettine KA, Morrey BF. Osteochondral fractures of the talus: a long-term follow-up. *J Bone Joint Surg.* 1987;69B:89-92.
4. Santrock RD, Buchanan MM, Lee TH, Berlet GC. Osteochondral lesions of the talus. *Foot Ankle Clin N Am.* 2003;8:73-90.
5. Paul J, Sagstetter A, Kriner M, et al. Donor-site morbidity after osteochondral autologous transplantation for lesions of the talus. *J Bone Joint Surg Am.* 2009;91:1683-1688.

How Do You Treat Chronic Achilles Tendinosis? When Do You Operate?

Steven A. Kodros, MD

Chronic Achilles tendinosis is a difficult and challenging clinical problem. It is characterized histologically by the presence of mucoid degeneration within the Achilles tendon. It is classified clinically by the location of the involvement: noninsertional (midsubstance) and insertional. Nonoperative management of Achilles tendinosis is similar regardless of the location of the involvement. First-line treatment includes the use of heel lifts in everyday shoe wear, nonsteroidal anti-inflammatory medication, periodic ice, and activity modification (most notably avoidance of uphill incline exercise). Use of a dorsiflexion night splint is also very helpful, particularly if the patient complains of startup pain. Perhaps most important is a home exercise program directed at eccentric strengthening exercises. Although immobilization can be considered, it is usually only of very limited usefulness except in cases of relatively acute onset of symptoms. If these initial efforts prove unsuccessful, then a brisement procedure can be considered (particularly for noninsertional Achilles tendinosis). This is usually done by our radiologists under ultrasound guidance. The diseased tendon is penetrated multiple times with a needle and small amounts of normal saline can be injected. This is felt to stimulate neovascularization within the tendon. The results are somewhat unpredictable (~ 60% to 80% good or excellent), but the risk is low and the recovery relatively quick. Extracorporeal shockwave treatment has also shown promising results (particularly for insertional Achilles tendinosis); however, insurance coverage for this is commonly denied. If nonoperative treatment efforts are exhausted, surgical intervention can be undertaken. However, patients should be cautioned that the recovery can be lengthy and the results somewhat unpredictable. Appropriate imaging studies to evaluate Achilles tendinosis include magnetic resonance imaging or musculoskeletal ultrasound. However, these are generally not necessary for conservative management.

Surgical treatment for noninsertional Achilles tendinosis generally involves débridement of the degenerative tendon. This is done through a longitudinal posteromedial or posterior incision placed over the thickened portion of the Achilles tendon. The tendon is

Figure 18-1. Intraoperative noninsertional Achilles tendinosis.

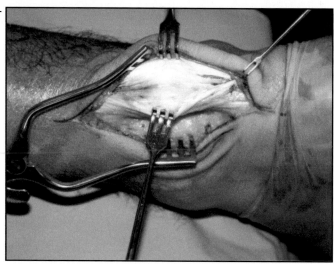

exposed and a longitudinal tenotomy is created within the Achilles tendon in line with its fibers (Figure 18-1).

Through this, the central core of the tendon is exposed and the areas of abnormal tendon can be débrided. If less than 50% or so of the tendon's cross-sectional area is resected, then a primary repair of the tenotomy incision is performed with a running monofilament suture. If more than 50% of the Achilles tendon is resected, then augmentation of the repair should be performed. (Preoperative imaging may help to predict this, but the ultimate determination should be based on the intraoperative findings.) Although a variety of different materials and grafts have been proposed for augmentation, I prefer to use the autogenous flexor hallucis longus (FHL) via a short harvest transferred to the calcaneal tuberosity (see the surgical technique described next). Postoperative management includes immobilization in a posterior splint nonweight bearing for 1 week followed by active range-of-motion exercises and weight bearing protected in a Controlled Ankle Movement (CAM) Walker boot for 6 weeks. After that, more aggressive supervised physical therapy with eccentric strengthening can be implemented.

For insertional Achilles tendinosis, surgical treatment with a limited débridement and excision of the Haglund's deformity has been described. However, this condition, particularly chronic calcific insertional Achilles tendinosis, is generally associated with more global involvement of the entire Achilles tendon insertion. As such, I prefer a more radical resection of the entire diseased Achilles tendon insertion (Figures 18-2 and 18-3).

If the patient has a gastrocnemius equinus contracture, then a gastrocnemius tendon recession is performed initially through a separate posteromedial incision proximally in the leg. The Achilles tendon is exposed through a longitudinal posteromedial incision and the insertion is then débrided. The posterior superior calcaneal tuberosity is decorticated and the Haglund's deformity, if present, is resected. Through the initial incision, the FHL is exposed by incising the deep crural fascia longitudinally anterior to the Achilles tendon. The FHL tendon is divided distally within the incision, being mindful of the neurovascular bundle medially. An eyelet containing trocar is then advanced from the superior aspect of the calcaneal tuberosity (just anterior to the insertion of the Achilles) antegrade out the plantar aspect of the heel. A 7-mm cannulated reamer is then used to

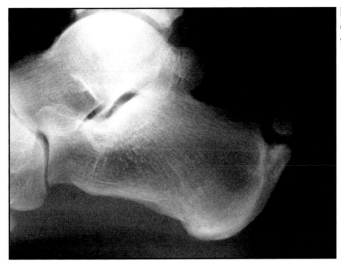

Figure 18-2. Preoperative x-ray of chronic calcific insertional Achilles tendinosis.

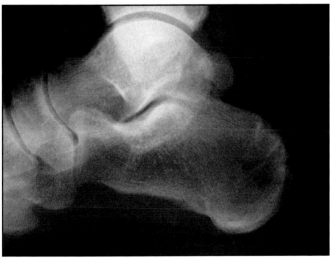

Figure 18-3. Postoperative x-ray status postdébridement of chronic calcific insertional Achilles tendinosis with FHL tendon transfer.

create a bone tunnel over this trocar. An absorbable grasping suture is then woven into the harvested FHL tendon and passed through to the bottom of the foot using the eyelet in the trocar. This suture is then used to assist in delivering the FHL tendon into the prepared bone tunnel and then to apply the appropriate tension on the FHL transfer. With this tension being maintained, the FHL tendon transfer is secured with a single 7-mm Bio-Tenodesis absorbable interference screw (Arthrex, Inc, Naples, FL). The absorbable tensioning suture is then trimmed flush with the plantar aspect of the heel. The remaining Achilles tendon is then reattached to the prepared posterior superior aspect of the calcaneal tuberosity using suture anchors or the Achilles SutureBridge (Arthrex, Inc). Finally, a side-to-side anastomosis of the FHL tendon transfer to the Achilles tendon is performed. Postoperative care includes immobilization in a posterior splint nonweight bearing for 3 weeks. After that, protection is continued in a CAM Walker boot, which is removed to perform periodic active range-of-motion exercises. Nonweight bearing is continued for a total of approximately 6 to 8 weeks postoperatively. Next, weight bearing

Figure 18-4. Intraoperative photo of calcaneal bone tunnel preparation for FHL transfer.

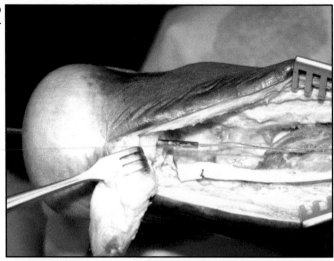

Figure 18-5. Intraoperative photo status post transfer of the FHL to the calcaneus.

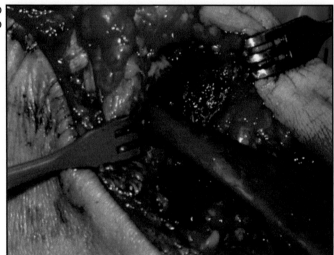

is advanced while protected in a CAM Walker boot. At approximately 12 weeks postoperatively, the CAM Walker boot is discontinued and more aggressive supervised physical therapy is implemented. Return to exercise and athletic participation can begin at 4 to 6 months postoperatively depending on the level and the recovery. It should be explained to the patient that it may take up to 1 to 2 years before the final results are achieved (Figures 18-4 and 18-5).

Suggested Readings

Den Hartog BD. Insertional Achilles tendinosis: pathogenesis and treatment. *Foot Ankle Clin N Am.* 2009;14(4):639-650.

Murphy GA. Surgical treatment of non-insertional Achilles tendonitis. *Foot Ankle Clin N Am.* 2009;14(4):652-661.

Young A, Redfern DJ. Simple method of local harvest and fixation of FHL in Achilles tendon reconstruction: technique tip. *Foot Ankle Int.* 2008;29(11):1148-1150.

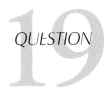

How Do I Know if I Should Transfer the Flexor Hallucis Longus or Do a Turn-Down or V-Y Lengthening for My Achilles Tendon Gap?

Donald R. Bohay, MD, FACS and Robert S. Marsh, DO

We have traditionally used a flexor hallucis longus (FHL) transfer over a V-Y lengthening regardless of the gap size. There are several reasons why we favor the FHL over the V-Y lengthening. One concern has been that advancement of the Achilles tendon more than 5 cm with the V-Y technique could ultimately weaken the musculotendinous unit.[1] We have not experienced a problem harvesting a long FHL tendon to make up for long gaps. Coull et al[2] performed a pedobarographic study on patients with an FHL transfer. Despite having weakness with hallux flexion, the patients did not report a functional weakness. Additionally, the V-Y tends to be a bulky transfer, which may bother the patients and result in a soft tissue problem at closure.

The FHL muscle is an in-phase muscle with the gastrocnemius-soleus complex during gait, thus providing a synergistic effect to the Achilles tendon during plantarflexion and gait. Finally, the FHL transfer is a relatively safe dissection as it avoids the neurovascular bundles associated with other tendon transfers such as the flexor digitorum longus (FDL; tibial nerve and artery) and the V-Y (sural nerve).[3]

We typically use a medial longitudinal incision along the Achilles tendon. Care is taken to make full thickness flaps, accepting a longer incision over a short one that would result in undue tension at the apex of the incision. The paratenon is incised in line with the skin incision. Often times, the diseased tendon involves multiple adhesions to the paratenon itself. Care is used to gently release the paratenon; typically, blunt dissection with a finger is all that is required. Débridement of the diseased tendon is then performed. The amount of débridement depends on the amount of fibromyxoid tissue present. I prefer removing as much of the diseased tendon needed to obtain healthier tissue or, as in the case presented, removing the segment entirely (Figure 19-1).

To harvest the FHL distally, a second incision is made at the plantar-medial border of the foot in line with the first metatarsal. There is frequently a cascade of veins along the

Figure 19-1. Exposure of calcaneus following débridement of achilles and excision of Haglund's deformity.

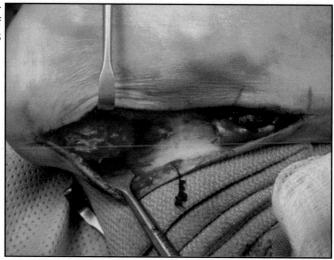

medial side of the foot that need to be ligated to help prevent postoperative hematoma formation. The abductor hallucis; flexor hallucis brevis; and the medial plantar artery, vein, and nerve are retracted plantar. At this point, there is typically a fibrous-fatty tissue overlying the sheaths of the FDL and FHL. Identification can be made by palpating the sheaths as the great toe is passively plantarflexed and dorsiflexed. Anatomically, the FHL tendon runs dorsal to the FDL distally and is harvested past the master knot of Henry (Figure 19-2). I do not routinely perform a tenodesis between the FHL and the FDL.

The deep compartment of the leg lies directly anterior to the Achilles tendon. The FHL tendon can be identified by pulling on the cut tendon and palpating the fascia overlying the tendon in the posterior compartment. The fascia of the posterior compartment is incised in-line with the tendon, and the tendon stump is retrieved into the posterior wound. Using a 6.5-mm drill, a medial to lateral hole is created in the calcaneus roughly 1 cm distal and 1 cm anterior to the insertion of the Achilles tendon. A small incision is made laterally to assist the passing of the FHL tendon medial to lateral (Figure 19-3).

The muscle belly of the FHL limits the extent of which the FHL is transferred into the calcaneus. The FHL is then tenodesed to itself distally and to the Achilles stump proximally with nonabsorbable sutures. The FHL belly is then sutured to the proximal stump of the remaining Achilles tendon. The paratenon is closed prior to wound closure and the patient is placed in a posterior, well-padded splint.

In our series of 17 patients with a 6- to 30-month follow-up, we reported no re-ruptures, tendinopathy recurrence, or wound dehiscence. Additionally, 75% were able to perform tip-toe stance on their operative side.[4] It should be noted that despite good results, the patient will experience some deficits of strength and range of motion with any repair of the Achilles tendon. It is difficult to predict the extent of deficit each patient may have, and it may be influenced by the time between repair, preoperative function, and quality of the repair.

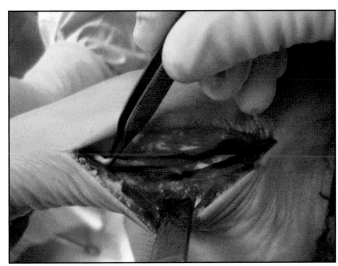

Figure 19-2. This figure shows the more dorsal location of the flexor hallucis longus in relation to the more plantar flexor digitorum longus.

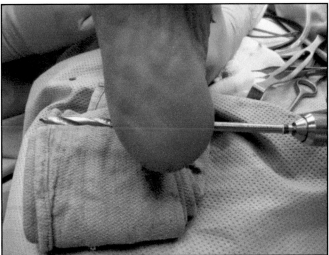

Figure 19-3. The transverse position of the drill in relationship to the calcaneus.

References

1. Myerson MS. Achilles tendon ruptures. *Instr Course Lect.* 1999;48:219-230.
2. Coull R, Flavin R, Stevens MM. Flexor hallucis longus tendon transfer: evaluation of postoperative morbidity. *Foot Ankle Int.* 2003;24:931-934.
3. Hansen ST. *Functional Reconstruction of the Foot and Ankle.* Philadelphia, PA: Lippincott, Williams & Wilkins; 2000:425-429.
4. Wilcox DK, Bohay DR, Anderson JG. Treatment of chronic Achilles tendon disorders with flexor hallucis longus tendon transfer/augmentation. *Foot Ankle Int.* 2000;21:1004-1010.

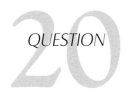

How Do You Treat a Haglund's Deformity That Does Not Have Any Changes Involving the Achilles Tendon?

W. Hodges Davis, MD

History

The presentation of patients with posterior heel pain provides an interesting diagnostic dilemma. The history-taking and demographics of this patient population are the most important tools in determining the proper management and treatment options. Most often, when patients present with posterior heel pain, it is activity related with a deformity (prominent heel bone; Figure 20-1). In the patient with a prominence in the posterior aspect of the calcaneus without Achilles tendon involvement, the activity-related pain is most often also shoe wear related. In addition, the pain is in a definitive spot each time the heel hurts. Patients with more Achilles tendinosis associated with their posterior heel pain will get radiation up the calf while patients with no Achilles involvement most often will have the pain isolated to the posterior heel. Most often, in these patients, the pain is on the posterolateral aspect of the heel, which is why it is often called a "pump bump," as this is where a woman's pump would rub on the back of the heel. My experience is that, in today's culture, the isolated pump bump is most often seen in young patients (younger than 30). Most of these patients rarely wear a pump and it seems athletic shoes are more often the culprit. The most common scenario is a young woman who is playing soccer or field hockey where the cleat actually rubs on the posterolateral heel. Occasionally, you will see it in a dancer, but a low-rise cleat is more common. There are some patients who describe a family history of this, and although it is not reported in the literature, my experience is that this type of prominence often runs in families.

Figure 20-1. Clinical picture of a prominent lateral ridge of the calcaneus or "pump bump."

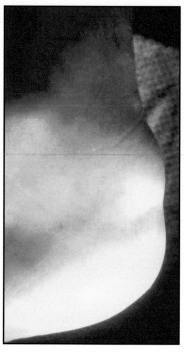

Physical Exam

Once a history is taken, it is important to perform a detailed physical examination. As in all hindfoot pathology, my routine requires a standing exam. Any asymmetric axial alignment issues should be noted. The most common deformity is mild symmetric intoeing. This variant of normal causes the running athlete to flare the heel out at end stance and can exacerbate a congenital prominence on the lateral calcaneus. It is then my routine to examine these patients in the prone position. This allows you to evaluate the calf for any asymmetry and the contralateral heel for any future potential problems, and it also allows you to evaluate the Achilles tendon in a more definitive manner. I will run my fingers along the Achilles tendon, as well as palpate the retro-Achilles space, to determine if there is any inflammation in that area. Most often, there is a callusing, swollen bursa, or other skin changes over this isolated prominent lateral calcaneal ridge. The prominent ridge is just lateral to the distal insertion point of the Achilles tendon. The calf is often symmetrical in size and the resting tension to the Achilles tendon is normal.

Radiographic Evaluation

The x-ray evaluation of these patients is fairly straightforward. I only require a standing lateral of the ankle and foot. This allows me to look at the anterior aspect of the ankle to determine if there is an equinus posture that predisposes to this lesion or some forefoot equinus that can create mild varus in the heel. At the same time, the evidence of any calcification in the Achilles tendon or calcification in and around the congenital calcaneal deformity is present. I rarely will draw the "Haglund's lines" as doing so does not provide any clinical benefits. There have been reports in the radiology literature that parallel lines can determine a diagnosis of a Haglund's deformity, although the clinical benefit is minimal. Magnetic resonance imaging (MRI) is not necessary if a careful physical examination is performed, although many patients come in with an MRI that shows a pristine Achilles tendon with minimal to no significant retro-Achilles inflammation. It is not unusual for an MRI to suggest edema in the calcaneus, most likely as a result of direct pressure.

Treatment

The predominant treatment mechanism for this patient population is nonoperative. There are a number of low profile pads that are available commercially that slide onto this area and can protect patients from their shoes. At the same time, some minimal shoe wear modifications such as changing either the dress shoes or athletic shoes by changing brands or techniques of padding and/or taping can give dramatic relief.

If the nonoperative management does not help, surgical management is fairly straight-forward. This is most often done with a lateral incision just below the actual bump. A subperiosteal dissection is made, exposing the posterior aspect of the calcaneus. I usually will expose the Achilles tendon and dissect it down to the insertion point without elevating the Achilles off of its insertion point. A fairly aggressive Haglund's resection is performed all the way across from lateral to medial and as far down as the distal insertional ridge. A power rasp is used to plane down the sharp edges of the lateral calcaneus. The determination of when the resection is adequate is made by direct finger palpation over the skin after it is rotated back over the bone rather than over the bone itself. Intraoperative x-ray is always done to confirm the resection margins. The prominence needs to be completely removed. With this patient population, I will usually place some bone wax on the bleeding bone that will decrease the incidence of a hematoma, which has been a reported complication.

Postoperative Care

In the postoperative period, the patient will be placed in a splint for 14 to 17 days to allow the wound to heal without complication. The sutures will be removed at that point, and a tall boot is used for another 2 to 3 weeks. Typically, by 6 weeks the patient is in a backless shoe and beginning to increase his or her activity. Rarely does he or she need formal physical therapy after this, and it just takes time for the swelling to resolve. Most patients will wear a commercially available silicone pad over the surgical area when wearing a closed-back shoe until about 4 months postoperatively to protect the scar.

The results with this surgery are encouraging. It is like, as we describe in our practices, old-fashioned orthopedics that you remove the pump and get the patients going, and they universally do well. The important points are proper diagnosis at the outset, nonoperative options first, and aggressive resection of the offending prominence.

MAGNETIC RESONANCE IMAGING SHOWS A PERONEUS TENDON TEAR. SHOULD I OPERATE?

Keith L. Wapner, MD

When evaluating magnetic resonance imaging (MRI) for injury to the peroneal tendons, it is important to look at both the sagittal and axial views. The axial views are often the most helpful in defining pathology. On axial images, the peroneal tendons should appear as low-signal-intensity structures posterior to the lateral malleolus. The peroneus brevis tendon generally is anteromedial to the peroneus longus tendon (Figure 21-1A). They then continue distally along the lateral wall of the calcaneus with the brevis dorsal and the longus plantar to the peroneal tubercle (Figure 21-1B). The brevis then inserts on the base of the fifth metatarsal and the longus travels under the cuboid toward the first metatarsal base. An os perineum bone or cartilage analog will be found at the point where the longus turns under the cuboid (Figure 21-2).

The peroneus brevis tendon is flat or mildly crescentic as it conforms to the shape of the retromalleolar groove, whereas the peroneus longus tendon appears globular in configuration (Figure 21-3). If there is increased signal intensity of the tendons, this is consistent with some type of tendon pathology (see Figure 21-3). It is first necessary to determine if the peroneus brevis, longus, or both tendons are involved (Figure 21-4). You also need to determine if there is a peroneus quartus tendon present (Figure 21-5). There may be associated subluxation of the tendon with no tendinopathy or there may be an associated longitudinal split tear of one or both peroneal tendons with or without significant surrounding synovitis. There can also be complete dislocation of the tendons (Figure 21-6). Once there is associated tendinosis, surgery would most likely be indicated. When there is involvement of both the peroneus longus and brevis, surgery is generally required.

The MRI evaluation must be correlated with the physical exam in determining the presence of subluxation of the tendons as an MRI is a static modality and subluxation may occur when the foot and ankle are in a position other than that demonstrated on the MRI. The MRI does, however, allow evaluation of the redundancy of the peroneal retinaculum as well as evaluation of the posterior border of the fibula. Identification of subluxation of

Figure 21-1. (A) Axial view of normal peroneal tendons. (B) Sagittal MRI of normal peroneal tendons.

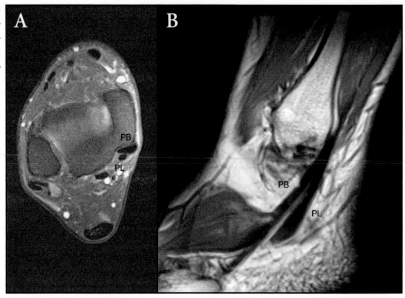

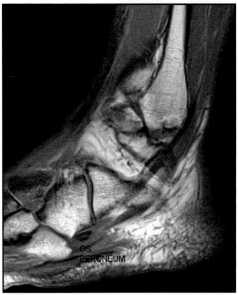

Figure 21-2. Sagittal MRI showing the os perineum at the level of the cuboid.

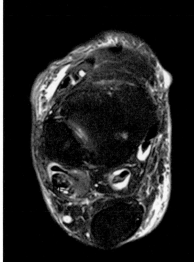

Figure 21-3. Axial MRI showing increased signal in the peroneus longus consistent with chronic tendinosis.

the tendon is critical as this is often the etiology of the split tears in the peroneus brevis tendon. Peroneal tendinosis often occurs as a secondary event to recurrent subluxation or secondary to an acute traumatic event (Figure 21-7). Unlike the posterior tibial tendon, peroneal tendon tears tend to be more longitudinal and amenable to primary repair when they are not associated with significant degenerative tendinosis. It becomes more difficult when there are tears of both tendons, especially if there is associated stenosis of the tendons within the peroneal sheath (Figure 21-8).

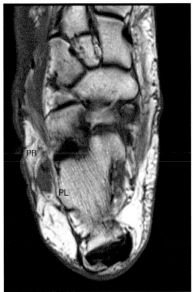

Figure 21-4. Axial MRI showing increased signal and size of both the peroneus brevis and longus consistent with tendinosis.

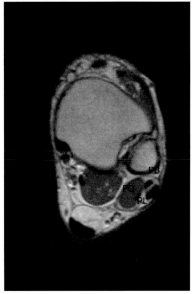

Figure 21-5. Axial MRI showing a peroneus quartus medial to the peroneus brevis and longus.

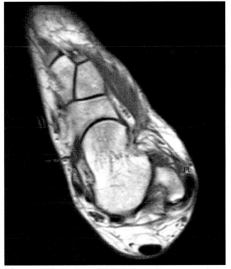

Figure 21-6. Axial MRI showing complete dislocation of the peroneus brevis and longus from behind the fibula with a convex posterior border of the fibula.

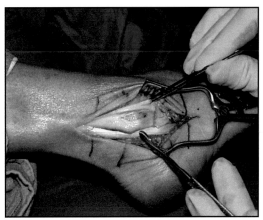

Figure 21-7. Intraoperative view of a tear of the peroneus brevis draped over the distal fibula.

In evaluating the MRI scan in conjunction with the physical examination, all possible components of surgery need to be identified. These include defining the areas where there is a longitudinal tear of the tendon or associated tendinosis, defining the area where there is subluxation of the tendon with redundancy of the peroneal retinaculum, or determining if the peroneal retinaculum is avulsed off its normal insertion off the posterior

Figure 21-8. Intraoperative view of tears of the peroneus brevis and longus and scarring within the peroneal sheath.

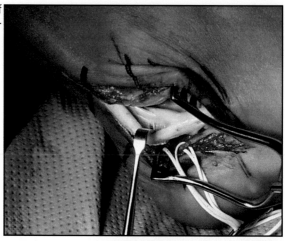

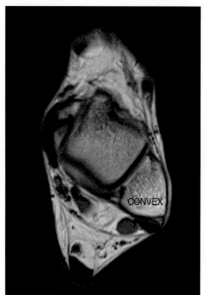

Figure 21-9. Axial MRI showing convex posterior border of the fibula.

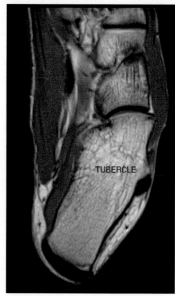

Figure 21-10. Axial MRI showing enlarged peroneal tubercle.

border of the fibula. You need to determine whether the posterior border of the fibula is concave or convex and thus contributing to the subluxation of the tendons (Figure 21-9). Evaluating the size of the peroneal tubercle is also important as this may be a cause of tearing of the peroneus longus secondary to impingement (Figure 21-10). The comprehensive plan should be adapted to address all of the abnormalities.

If the MRI demonstrates a small isolated split tear of the peroneus brevis or isolated stenosis, it may be possible to treat this nonoperatively. Once there is a significant tear, especially with associated tenosynovitis, operative intervention with débridement and repair of the tendon will generally be necessary (Figure 21-11). With split tears of both tendons, operative intervention should be considered. The peroneus longus may be torn at the level of the peroneal tubercle in cases where the tubercle is hypertrophic, and the tubercle may need to be débrided at the time of repair.

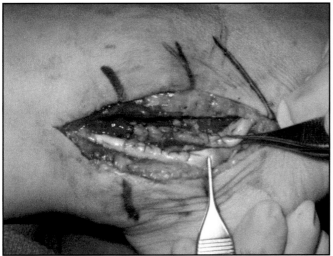

Figure 21-11. Intraoperative view of repaired peroneus brevis and longus tears.

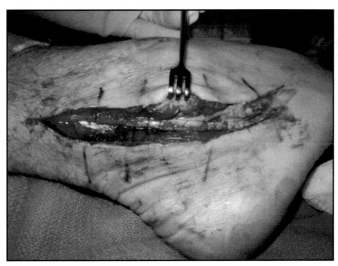

Figure 21-12. Intraoperative view of peroneus brevis anastomosed to peroneus longus for repair of tears of both tendons.

When subluxation or dislocation of the tendons is found, this must be addressed surgically to restore the normal tracking of the tendons. The presence of redundancy or avulsion of the peroneal retinaculum can be identified and must be repaired. If the posterior border of the fibula is convex, a bony procedure should be included to deepen the groove for the peroneal tendons. This can be done in conjunction with a repair of the tendinosis, if present.

Once peroneal tendinosis is present, operative intervention is required.[1,2] The extent of tendinosis will determine if primary repair is possible. If not severe, débridement of the tendon and tabularization can be attempted. If one tendon is involved and the other is normal, excision of the involved segment with anastomosis above and below may be required (Figure 21-12). When there is severe involvement of both tendons, it is more problematic and this may indicate that a tendon transfer needs to be considered. If the peroneal sheath is intact, this can be done as a primary flexor hallucis longus transfer. If there has been previous surgery, severe disruption, or stenosis of the peroneal sheath, a staged procedure using a Hunter rod and a later flexor hallucis transfer can be performed.[3]

With any peroneal pathology, the posture of the foot needs to be assessed. The presence of a varus posture of the calcaneus either from a primary or acquired cavus foot may need to be addressed. This cannot be assessed by MRI and needs to be assessed on physical exam and standing, weight-bearing x-ray.

The presence of any underlying neurologic condition that may predispose to peroneal weakness, acquired cavus or cavovarus deformity, or post-traumatic neurologic injury must be identified and considered in conjunction with the MRI findings. Correction of the underlying foot deformity may be an integral part of the repair of the foot and ankle to assure that the repair of the tendon is protected.

References

1. Mizel MS, Michelson JD, Wapner KL. *Diagnosis and Treatment of Peroneus Brevis Injury Foot and Ankle Clinics: Tendon Injury and Reconstruction.* Vol 1(2). Philadelphia, PA: W.B. Saunders; 1996.
2. Heckman DS, Reddy S, Pedowitz D, Wapner K, Parekh SG. Operative treatment for peroneal tendon disorders. *J Bone Joint Surg.* 2008;90A(2):404-418.
3. Wapner KL, Parekh SG, Pedowitz DI, Chao W, Hecht PJ. Reconstruction of chronic peroneal tendon ruptures with staged Hunter rods and a flexor hallucis longus transfer. *Tech Foot Ankle Surg.* 2005;4(3):202-206.

How Do You Manage Ankle Arthritis With Minimal Arthritic Changes on Radiographs?

Pradeep Kodali, MD and Anand Vora, MD

When treating patients with ankle arthritis with minimal arthritic changes on radiographs, it is always important to consider the underlying cause(s) of the condition. Primary ankle osteoarthritis is rare. More commonly, ankle arthritis is a result of post-traumatic injury. Inflammatory arthropathies, neuropathic conditions, and other rare conditions such as hemophilia or tuberculosis should also be considered. Lastly, and perhaps most importantly, periarticular instability conditions such as lateral ankle ligament instability with or without underlying bony malalignment require recognition.

In evaluating radiographs, it is critical for films to be weight bearing. The arthritic involvement of the tibiotalar joint on anteroposterior and mortise views should be differentiated as symmetric and diffuse intra-articular involvement from asymmetric joint involvement. Focal localized arthritic conditions as a result of traumatic or atraumatic conditions, including osteochondral lesions, should also be differentiated from diffuse symmetric involvement of the joint. The presence of loose bodies should also be appreciated. Lateral radiographs in early arthritic conditions will demonstrate anterior osteophytes with preservation of the central and posterior portion of the joint (Figure 22-1A). A medial oblique lateral view may be necessary to better identify the presence of anterior tibial osteophytes.

Treatment of symptomatic arthritis with minimal arthritic changes should begin with activity modification, weight loss in obese patients, and nonsteroidal anti-inflammatory agents. In conditions associated with soft tissue instability (ie, lateral ankle instability), physical therapy may be considered for strengthening of the lateral restraints. Impact activities such as jumping sports should be avoided and emphasis placed on activities such as swimming and bicycling. Intra-articular injection of corticosteroids can be used, albeit with variable clinical efficacy, if patients have an acute flare or if refractory to other measures. Viscosupplementation with hyaluron injections has been reported; however, it is not FDA approved and has not been an effective treatment in our clinical experience.

Figure 22-1. (A) Pre-operative view showing anterior impinging osteophyte (arrow). (B) Postoperative view after resection (arrow).

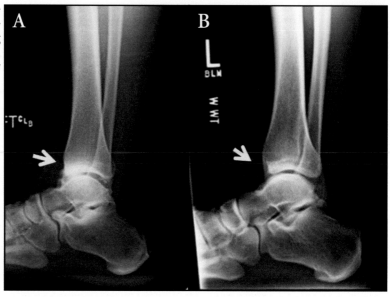

Footwear modifications or brace application can be very effective and are the mainstay of conservative treatment. A rocker-bottom sole or a solid ankle cushion heel can improve gait and reduce pain. We have found that the use of commercially available over-the-counter shoes, which incorporate such modifications in their design, have lead to an improved patient acceptance and compliance. Custom orthotics may be useful in an attempt to accommodate asymmetric load on the ankle. An ankle-foot orthotic or a lace-up ankle gauntlet brace support is often very effective in immobilizing the ankle and/or correcting malalignment of an arthritic joint when tolerated by patients.

Operative treatment options for persistent pain are dependant on the specific arthritic findings. An arthroscopic treatment is the preferred option for loose bodies, impinging osteophytes, impinging synovium, and localized chondral defects. We like to use an ankle distraction device for all arthroscopic procedures. An initial medial portal is made between the tibialis anterior and medial malleolus at the level of the joint. An initial skin incision is made and, using a hemostat, the subcutaneous tissue is bluntly dissected to capsule. The hemostat is then used to penetrate the capsule. This technique of creating portals minimizes injury to the neurovascular structures in the area. The lateral portal is created in similar fashion under direct visualization lateral to the peroneus tertius. A complete arthroscopy is performed addressing any chondral lesions, removing loose bodies, and débriding anterior osteophytes (most commonly located on the anterolateral tibia). A successful resection of the anterior tibial osteophyte usually can be performed arthroscopically; however, a mini-arthrotomy can be used for complete resection if necessary (Figure 22-1B). Intraoperative fluoroscopic lateral and oblique views are useful to assure complete arthroscopic osteophyte resection. Arthroscopy is not indicated for advanced arthritis, marked fibrosis, and severe deformity. It should be noted that in such cases, arthroscopy might not only fail to provide relief but rather further exacerbate symptoms.

A brief discussion on treatment of focal osteochondral defects should be included in the management of arthritis with minimal radiographic changes. These focal defects can

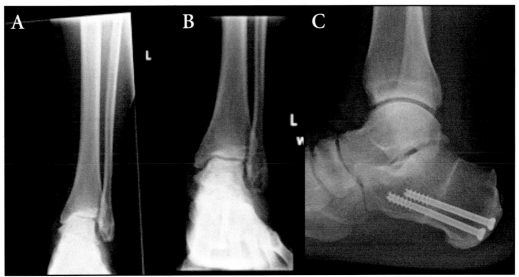

Figure 22-2. (A) Preoperative view of a patient with lateral ligament instability, arthritis, and varus deformity. (B) Anteroposterior view after lateral ligament reconstruction and calcaneal osteotomy. (C) Lateral view after lateral ligament reconstruction and calcaneal osteotomy.

alter the mechanical forces of the adjacent normal cartilage, thus advancing cartilage wear over time. Osteochondral defects are most commonly post-traumatic and often associated with ankle sprains or ankle fractures. If there is evidence of an osteochondral lesion with or without a loose body, then an ankle arthroscopy is considered. Lesions that are <1.5 cm^2 in diameter as measured by arthroscopic evaluation are treated with débridement and microfracture with the expectation of healing with fibrocartilage. We also consider arthroscopy with débridement and microfracture as first-line treatment for larger lesions if no cystic changes are present in the talar body. Lesions between 1.5 to 2.5 cm^2 can be treated with mosaicplasty autograft technique with donor tissue obtained from the ipsilateral nonweight-bearing portion of the distal femur. However, our preference is to use matched fresh frozen talar allograft for any lesions >1.5 cm^2 to avoid donor site morbidity and for any lesion that has failed arthroscopic débridement and microfracture.

Lastly, treating the underlying problem causing ankle arthritis is key to preventing progression to advanced radiographic and clinical changes. For ankle instability, a lateral ligamentous reconstruction is necessary to realign and stabilize the ankle. We have found that in patients who have such severe instability that arthritis has already occurred, an anatomic reconstruction technique such as a modified Broström procedure alone is not sufficient. Most patients require a more advanced reconstructive procedure such as an allograft lateral ankle ligament reconstruction or peroneal augmentation procedure to obtain soft tissue stability. In addition to correcting the soft tissue component of malalignment, bony correction with extra-articular osteotomy procedures of the calcaneus, tibia, and occasionally the first metatarsal are also necessary to correct the underlying foot deformity (Figure 22-2). This is the case in patients requiring a cavus foot reconstruction.

In patients with post-traumatic ankle arthritic conditions, addressing the site of malunion, if any, can be beneficial in preventing further progression of the arthritic condition of the ankle. For example, in patients with tibial malunion, an osteotomy is performed at the center of rotation of angulation using standard principles to realign the appropriate weight-bearing axis. In patients with malunion and shortening of the fibula, a lengthening osteotomy of the fibula with rotational correction and reconstruction of the syndesmosis to restore the normal tibiotalar relationship may prevent the development of further arthrosis.

Finally, osteotomies of the distal tibia or calcaneus are useful not only to correct bony malunion or underlying foot deformities, but are independently powerful in redistributing forces across the tibiotalar joint in cases where such deformity may not exist. For example, in patients with osteoarthritis of intermediate grade characterized by a varus deformity and anterior opening of the tibiotalar joint and medial malleolar hypoplasia, an opening wedge low tibial osteotomy is considered. In a similar fashion, a lateralizing calcaneal osteotomy in patients with a varus deformity of the ankle may be an effective adjunct to redistribute the forces and the level of the tibiotalar joint to the more normal portion of the joint. The specific techniques of such osteotomies are beyond the scope of this chapter.

Ankle arthritis with minimal radiographic changes is a difficult problem. Every effort to avoid surgery is made as there is no clear, reliable surgical technique. Treatment should be individualized to underlying pathology and deformity. Even so, long-term studies have not shown that any surgical technique will prevent progression to advanced arthritis.

Suggested Readings

Chou L, Coughlin M, Hansen S, et al. Osteoarthritis of the ankle: the role of arthroplasty. *J Am Acad Orthop Surg.* 2008;16(5):249-259.

Stone JW. Osteochondral lesions of the talar dome. *J Am Acad Orthop Surg.* 1996;4:63-73.

Takakura Y, Tanaka Y, Kumal T, Tamai S. Low tibial osteotomy for osteoarthritis of the ankle. *J Bone Joint Surg Br.* 1995;77-B:50-54.

Thomas R, Daniels T. Ankle arthritis. *J Bone Joint Surg Am.* 2003;85:923-936.

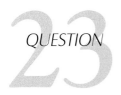

QUESTION

WILL AN ANKLE ARTHROSCOPY AND REMOVAL OF BONE SPURS HELP ME?

Armen S. Kelikian, MD

The advent of ankle arthroscopy has eliminated the need for open arthrotomy for a number of disorders ranging from loose bodies, soft tissue impingement, osteochondral lesions, and even some arthrodesis. The critical question in regard to the patient described above is to determine if the lesion is simple impingement or osteoarthritis. Impingement spurs are common from repetitive microtrauma from forced dorsiflexion or capsular avulsion from plantarflexion. The chief complaint is difficulty with dorsiflexion range of motion—squatting, pushing off, running, or going up or down stairs. Symptoms are of a gradual onset and usually do not prevent the patient from attempting to perform activities. Complaints are not typically of pain but of a mechanical obstruction or block. Classically, the physical exam will show decreased ankle range of motion, particularly in dorsiflexion compared to the opposite limb. This may further be accentuated by having the patient attempt to squat and noting how the affected heel will rise off the ground earlier than the opposite side. Pain may be elicited with palpation anteriorly over the joint line and the examination may be able to palpate the osteophyte. Limited dorsiflexion may also be due to gastrocnemius contracture, which can be assessed during the exam. Patients will describe tightness in their Achilles versus an anterior joint line mechanical obstruction while attempting maximal dorsiflexion (see Question 12).

Diagnostic assessment should include weight-bearing anteroposterior and lateral radiographs. On the lateral view, the angle between the distal tip of the tibia and talus should be greater than 60 degrees. A computed tomography or magnetic resonance imaging scan can be an adjunct in helping to determine if there is adequate cartilage remaining to afford débridement. Impingement spurs are usually anterolateral but can be anteromedial or central. While the spurs are more common at the distal anterior aspect of the tibia, there can be a corresponding "kissing" lesion on the talar neck. Scranton and McDermott have classified these from Grades I through IV. Grade IV lesions were not as amenable to arthroscopic resection (Table 23-1). However, if radiographs show a well-maintained joint space combined with a physical exam of isolated anterior

Table 23-1

Grade of Spur Formation

Grade I	Synovial impingement up to 3-mm tibial span
Grade II	Tibial span >3 mm
Grade III	Significant tibial exostosis with or without fragmentation; secondary spur formation on dorsum of talus
Grade IV	Pantalocrural arthritic destruction (not candidates for arthroscopic débridement)

Adapted from Scranton PE Jr, McDermott JE. Anterior tibiotalar spurs: a comparison of open versus arthroscopic debridement. *Foot Ankle.* 1992;13:125-129.

Figure 23-1. (A) Anterior osteophyte with tibiotalar angle more than 60 degrees. (B) Postresection.

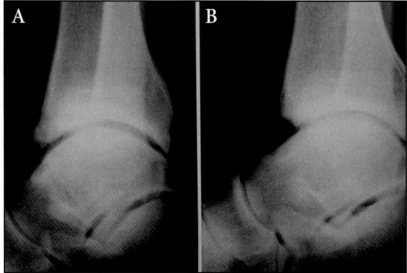

tenderness, then there may be a role for arthroscopic débridement (Figure 23-1). This patient population will do well with ankle arthroscopy and removal of anterior osteophyte provided they do not have more global arthritic changes. The preoperative discussion needs to be thorough and include expectations about the surgery. Although activity-related pain will usually decrease, the range of motion may not change significantly.[1]

The second population is those spurs seen due to osteoarthritis. In cases of osteoarthritis, patients will have more typical arthritic symptoms such as morning and start-up pain and stiffness, weather-related changes, and more chronic pain in all weight-bearing phases of the gait cycle. Symptoms are usually gradual in onset and are commonly associated with a previous history of trauma. Weight-bearing radiographs in this patient population will typically show more global and diffuse joint space narrowing. While these patients may show evidence of significant anterior osteophytes, their radiographs are typically more globally involved. These patients, similar to patients with knee osteoarthritis, do not

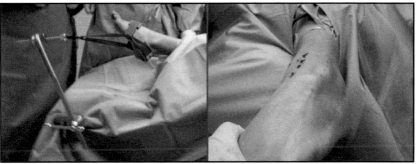

Figure 23-2. Arthroscopy setup.

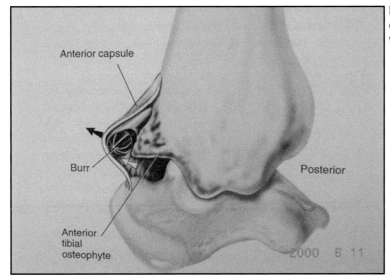

Figure 23-3. Anterior osteophyte right ankle with burr.

do well with a simple ankle arthroscopy and débridement. Unless symptoms are focalized or there is discrete evidence of loose bodies, arthroscopy should not be attempted.

Ankle Arthroscopy

If nonoperative measures such as heel lifts, nonsteroidal anti-inflammatory drugs, gastrocnemius soleus stretches, and intra-articular steroid injections have failed, then resection may be indicated. Noninvasive distraction and inflow are needed. Standard anteromedial and anterolateral portals should suffice (Figure 23-2). Visualization of the anterior and inferior extent of the spurs needs to be exposed using a 3.5- or 4-mm aggressive oscillating shaver to remove the anterior capsule off the distal tibia. The bone may be burred (4 mm) by shaving in a single direction (Figures 23-3 through 23-5). I often find that an aggressive resection is required. Intra-arthroscopy assessment of the resection is typically less than what the radiographs will show. A lateral radiograph ensures complete resection at the end of the procedure. My goal intraoperatively is 5 degrees of dorsiflexion motion. Intra-articular assessment with the ankle in maximal dorsiflexion

Figure 23-4. Right ankle using 3.5-mm aggressive shaver to débride the anterolateral tibial impingement spur.

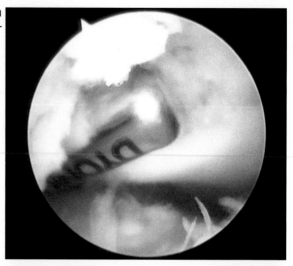

Figure 23-5. Anterior distal tibia after osteophyte removal.

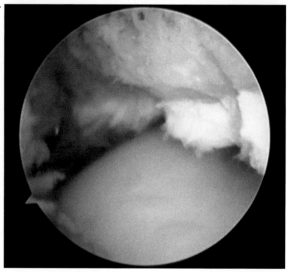

with direct visualization is performed; further anterior bony resection is performed versus consideration for a posterior procedure. After adequate anterior decompression has been confirmed and ankle dorsiflexion is still not 5 degrees past neutral, then a Strayer gastrocnemius recession should be considered.

Postoperative Protocol

Portal sites are sutured, a sterile dressing applied, and a 3-sided plaster splint is applied. Nonweight bearing of the affected limb is ordered. The dressing and sutures are removed at 7 to 10 days postoperatively. Progressive weight bearing is commenced. If a Strayer recession was performed, a Controlled Ankle Motion walker is used for an additional

2 weeks. Eccentric calf strengthening and gastrocsoleus stretches are emphasized. Return to sports can be at 6 to 10 weeks postoperatively. This is usually delayed an additional 4 to 6 weeks if a Strayer procedure was performed.

Reference

1. Ferkel RD, Cheng JC. Ankle and subtalar arthroscopy. In: Kelikian A, ed. *Operative Treatment of the Foot and Ankle.* Stamford, CT: Appleton & Lange; 1999:321-350.

I Have a 63-Year-Old Patient Who Had an Ankle Fracture 20 Years Ago and Is Ready for a Major Procedure Now. Should I Perform an Ankle Arthrodesis or Should I Refer Her to Someone for a Total Ankle Arthroplasty? What Are Your Criteria for a Total Ankle Arthroplasty?

Gregory C. Berlet, MD and Jaymes D. Granata, MD

Symptomatic ankle arthritis is a progressively disabling disease that can adversely affect both mobility and overall general health. As opposed to the hip or the knee, primary idiopathic arthritis of the ankle is relatively rare. The majority of patients with ankle arthritis report a history of ankle trauma. Inciting events range from isolated or recurrent ankle sprains to more traumatic fractures of the talus, malleoli, or tibial plafond. Post-traumatic arthritis is estimated to account for 79.5% of the total cases of ankle arthritis, compared to 1.6% and 9.8% for the hip and knee, respectively.[1] The traumatic etiology leads to an overall younger patient population with arthritis and represents a significant financial burden. Lost productivity and direct medical costs of treatment for lower extremity post-traumatic arthritis account for approximately 11.8 billion dollars annually in the United States.[1]

The primary goals of treatment for ankle arthritis are to alleviate pain and maintain or restore mobility. Conservative management includes nonsteroidal anti-inflammatory medications, bracing, and shoe modification. Despite these conservative measures, the progressive nature of ankle arthritis will lead many patients to eventually seek surgical consultation. In the early stages, arthroscopic débridement may be considered. Similar to the knee, generalized arthritis of the ankle does not respond well to arthroscopic débridement in the long term. Arthroscopy for ankle arthritis should be limited to loose body

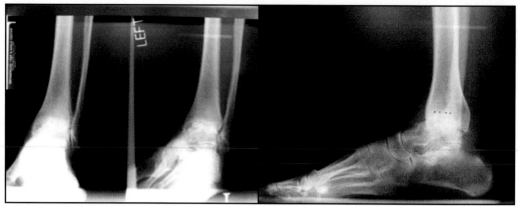

Figure 24-1. Standing 3 views of the ankle demonstrating isolated tibiotalar arthritis with minimal deformity.

removal. With advanced-stage, generalized arthritis of the ankle, there are 2 main surgical treatment options: ankle fusion and total ankle arthroplasty (TAA). The decision of which option to use remains a topic of much debate.

We still consider ankle fusion to be the gold standard treatment for ankle arthritis. For patients with a history of ankle infection, Charcot neuroarthropathy, poor circulation, and an inadequate or compromised soft tissue envelope, it is the only surgical option that we will offer. Fusion may also be more appropriate for manual laborers and those patients with an active lifestyle.

Ankle fusion is not a perfect procedure for all patients. As with any fusion surgery, there is a risk of nonunion, although with modern surgical techniques and biologic augmentation, nonunion rates are decreasing. Immobilizing the ankle joint adversely affects gait and increases energy consumption. Progression of adjacent joint arthritis is also a concern because fusion of the ankle increases the stress distribution to the distal joints in the foot.

To maintain motion in the ankle joint and avoid the drawbacks of fusion, TAA was introduced in the 1970s. Unfortunately, the first-generation implants and surgical techniques led to dismal results. The implants and surgical techniques have since been refined, leading to a renewed interest in TAA. A recent prospective randomized trial between ankle fusion and TAA with the Scandinavian total ankle replacement found that the TAA patients had equivalent pain relief and improved function as compared to the patients with a fusion at an average 24-month follow up.[2]

Our criteria for TAA is based on the patient's age, weight, activity level, amount of deformity, and tolerance for risk. We consider an ideal candidate to be healthy, not overweight, over the age of 60 years old, less active, with isolated tibiotalar arthritis, and with less than 20 degrees of valgus deformity. Our evaluation after a thorough history and physical exam includes weight-bearing anteroposterior, mortise, and lateral x-rays to evaluate the overall alignment and amount of deformity (Figure 24-1).

We use the standard anterior approach to the ankle for TAA. The surgical technique depends on the type of implant used. Regardless of the implant, appropriate coronal and sagittal plane alignment is essential to achieve the best range of motion and implant longevity (Figure 24-2).

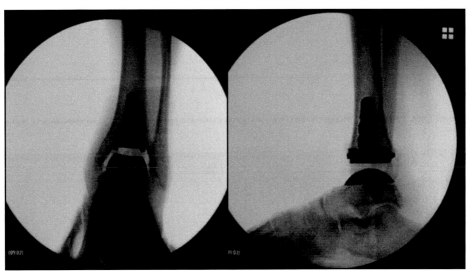

Figure 24-2. Intraoperative fluoroscopy verifying excellent coronal and sagittal plane alignment.

The indications for TAA are expanding to include patients with increased deformity and associated pathology. TAA is being combined with adjacent joint fusion procedures and ligament reconstructions. There are also reports of successful TAA in patients with a history of avascular necrosis of the talus as well as conversions of ankle fusions to TAA. Although we have very encouraging short- and intermediate-term results comparing fusion to TAA, the debate continues as to which treatment is best in the long term.

References

1. Brown TD, Johnston RC, Saltzmann CL, Marsh JL, Buckwalter JA. Posttraumatic osteoarthritis: a first estimate of incidence, prevalence, and burden of disease. *J Orthop Trauma*. 2006;20:739-744.
2. Saltzmann CL, Mann RA, Ahrens JE, et al. Prospective controlled trial of STAR total ankle replacement versus ankle fusion: initial results. *Foot Ankle Int*. 2009;30:579-596.

SECTION IV

SPORTS

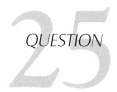

AN 18-YEAR-OLD MALE SOCCER PLAYER HAS DISLOCATING PERONEAL TENDONS. HOW WOULD YOU TREAT THIS?

Simon Lee, MD and Robert R. L. Gray, MD

In the setting of a recent acute traumatic episode of subluxation, a trial of nonoperative therapy (including abstinence from sports) and bracing, splinting, or casting of the ankle in a position of slight plantarflexion and inversion may be considered. This has been reported to provide relief to some patients and eliminate future instability if the superficial retinaculum is allowed to heal in an anatomic and functional position. Careful range of motion therapy should be initiated to prevent stiffness and an equines contracture. However, due to the prolonged period of immobilization and reported incidence as high as 50% of continued recurrent dislocations, I typically advocate repair to most patients.

While nonoperative treatment may be considered in instances of an acute peroneal tendon dislocation/subluxation, there is no indication for nonoperative treatment of the recurrent symptomatic subluxor. This is a mechanical problem that cannot be treated by physical therapy or bracing. In fact, physical therapy will often aggravate this condition with most strengthening and proprioceptive exercises intensifying the subluxation. Additionally, prolonged chronic subluxation will ultimately result in damage to the peroneal tendons. Avoidance of provocative maneuvers is usually not a viable option for the active patient.

In addressing the recurrent subluxor, it is important to understand the rarity of the condition as well as the frequency of missed or delayed diagnosis. Nearly 40% of these patients are incorrectly diagnosed as ankle sprains.[1] In my practice, any patient who has a "typical" ankle sprain with complaints of a "popping or snapping" sensation or without improvement in 4 to 6 weeks and worsening of their pain with physical therapy should be seriously evaluated for subtle chronic peroneal subluxation. These patients tend to be extremely frustrated due to the lack of a definitive diagnosis as well as the prolonged time and effort they have put into their recovery without improvement.

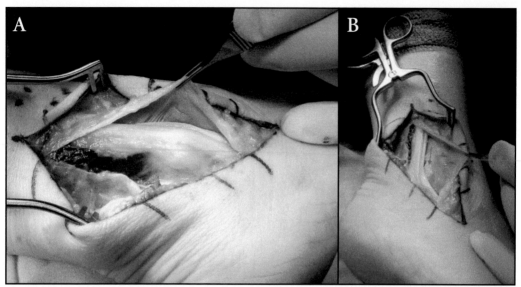

Figure 25-1. (A) Intraoperative photograph showing immediate visualization of the peroneal tendons upon incision of the peroneal flexor retinaculum versus the lateral border and periosteum of the fibula. Also note the amount of muscle from the peroneal brevis present at this level. (B) The same intraoperative photograph as in A with the peroneals reduced and also showing the avulsion of the retinaculum and periosteum of the fibula (arrow) forming a false pouch (arrow heads) that the peroneals were entrapped within.

As opposed to patients with classical ankle sprains with tenderness over the anterior aspect of the distal fibula, peroneal subluxors will have tenderness mainly over the posterior fibula. These patients often develop an apprehension sign to the provocative maneuver of resisted eversion and dorsiflexion. This can be accentuated by applying an anteriorly directed force to the tendons with the examiner's thumb. A version of the relocation test may be elicited if the patient's apprehension is relieved by direct pressure on the posterior edge of the fibula. In advanced cases, the tendons may be chronically dislocated and adherent to the lateral border of the fibula (Figure 25-1). Additionally, some patients may be able to voluntarily dislocate the tendons. In most patients, however, this often requires general anesthesia, much like a pivot-shift test in the knee.

Radiographs of the ankle may reveal a "fleck" sign posterolaterally in the distal fibula, indicating an avulsion of the superficial peroneal retinaculum (Figure 25-2). Magnetic resonance imaging (MRI) is the imaging modality of choice in evaluating these patients. Peroneal tendon tears, tears in the sheath, and fibular anatomy can be appreciated. Occasionally, the tendons can be seen to lie outside of the fibular groove or relative subluxation of the tendons within the sheath. Additionally, the depth of the peroneal groove can be assessed (Figure 25-3). Fluid within the sheath on T2 sequences can also be an indirect indicator of subluxation. Some authors have described obtaining an MRI with the foot in dorsiflexion to elicit the pathology. However, this is not reliably obtained, especially when patients are referred in with imaging already completed. Dynamic ultrasound may also be helpful, but it is operator dependent and not usually more sensitive than careful examination.

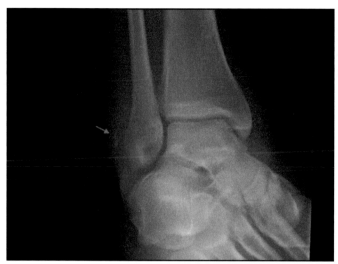

Figure 25-2. Oblique radiograph of the ankle showing the subtle "fleck" sign indicative of a superficial peroneal retinaculum avulsion injury.

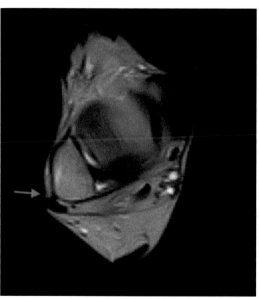

Figure 25-3. MRI image showing the peroneal tendons lateral to the fibula (arrow) at the level of the ankle mortise. Also note the lack of concavity (arrow heads) of the posterior fibula at this level.

I employ a multifactorial approach to surgical management. Understand that although numerous anatomic variables contributing to subluxation have been identified, it is difficult if not impossible to isolate a single causative factor in a given patient. Because all potential etiologies at each surgery are addressed, the patient has the best opportunity for symptom resolution with little to no added morbidity.

The anatomy of the peroneal groove, the overlying superficial peroneal retinaculum, and the contents of the peroneal compartment must be understood in planning the operation. The 3 basic components are the peroneal tendons within the groove, the sheath overlying it, and the groove itself.

First, I address the tendons within the groove. Initial inspection of the tendons should be performed to identify any intrinsic damage to the peroneals. The brevis tendon may take on a flattened morphology, which can contribute to subluxation. If needed, I will

Figure 25-4. Intraoperative photograph showing the peroneal tendons relocated posterior to the fibula. The peroneus brevis has also been tubularized. Also note the avulsion of the peroneal tendon sheath and periosteum from the posterior edge of the fibula.

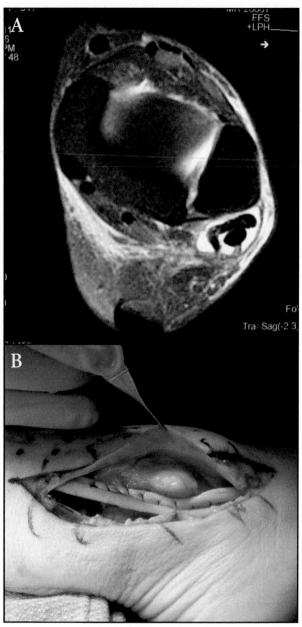

"tubularize" this tendon by running an absorbable whipstitch through the edges to draw them together (Figure 25-4). Additional evaluation of any mass-occupying effects in the tendon sheath should be addressed. An anomalous peroneus quartus or low-lying muscle on the peroneus brevis may be present and both must be excised. The peroneal tubercle should be evaluated as well since it may require excision.

Although the depth of the fibular groove is of questionable importance in causing subluxation, I routinely employ an indirect groove-deepening approach as described by Mendicino et al (Figure 25-5).[2] Using sequentially larger drill bits, the fibula is drilled

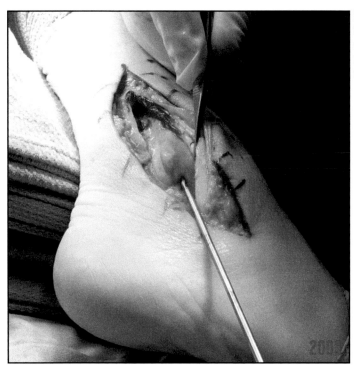

Figure 25-5. Note the indirect technique with use of a small drill bit to begin the distal intramedullary starting point in the fibula.

retrograde from the tip, approximately 4 to 5 cm into the bone, using the drill as a side-cutting reamer to remove bone from behind the fibular groove cartilage. Placing the operator's other index finger on the groove while drilling helps to judge the amount of bone resected and prevents breakthrough. After a large enough drill has been used, a curette can be introduced to provide a more tactile and controlled resection. The groove is then impacted using a flat bone tamp padded with a sponge. Ideally, 4 to 5 mm of deepening is desired. If the deepening is adequate, the tendons will not subluxate with dorsiflexion and eversion, even before the sheath is repaired.

Several other techniques such as fixing a bone block with screws or elevating the cartilage flap of the groove and directly removing the subchondral bone have been described. These techniques are more technically difficult and seem to cause more scarring due to the loss of the smooth sheath posteriorly. I have never found the indirect groove technique to fail.

The lateral border of the fibula should also be denuded to allow the repaired periosteum and retinaculum to adhere securely. Lastly, the peroneal sheath is repaired to the cartilage flap on the posterior fibula using interrupted nonabsorbable sutures in a pants-over-vest fashion. The knots are buried so as to not be prominent in this subcutaneous location, and the superficial retinaculum is repaired using interrupted absorbable suture.

Drains are not routinely needed and the leg is splinted in slight equinus and inversion to protect the repair. The patient is nonweight bearing for 2 weeks and gently progressed to weight bearing in a Controlled Ankle Movement boot. Avoidance of resisted dorsiflexion and eversion should be implemented for 6 to 8 weeks. Sporting activity is restricted for 3 months.

References

1. Dombek MF, Lamm BM, Saltrick K, Mendicino RW, Catanzariti AR. Peroneal tendon tears: a retrospective review. *J Foot Ankle Surg.* 2003;42(5):250-258.
2. Mendicino RW, Orsini RC, Whitman SE, Catanzariti AR. Fibular groove deepening for recurrent peroneal subluxation. *J Foot Ankle Surg.* 2001;40(4):252-263.

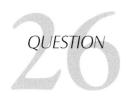

How Would You Treat a 22-Year-Old Professional Ballet Dancer With an Os Trigonum and Fluid Around Her Flexor Hallucis Longus Tendon Sheath Seen on Magnetic Resonance Imaging?

W. Hodges Davis, MD

History

The first thing that is important to define when a "professional" ballet dancer presents to your office is exactly what level of dance they are professional in. There are several levels of dance, and all are legitimate activities and are important for that particular dancer. The question that must be answered in a professional ballet dancer is how professional? How many weeks a year does she dance professionally, and does she have other jobs in addition to dance? Does the dancer have another job to supplement her income that does not involve dance? A full-time professional dancer is significantly more motivated, and the rehabilitation necessary to come back from any serious injury requires "professional" motivation. Hamilton et al reported that the postoperative functional results in flexor hallucis longus (FHL) tendinitis patients were significantly better in dancers who were professionals.[1] Secondly, the determination of what discipline of dance they are practicing is important. In addition, women and men have different types of injuries and dance requirements. A classical ballet dancer who is a female will be dancing en pointe, and because of that will have a unique stress on the posterior aspect of her ankle and her FHL. Classical ballet is the only dance regimen that requires the dancer to go en pointe, and females are the only dancers who go en pointe. The reality of pointe dancing is the FHL is required to allow the dancer to get on her toes. If the dancer is doing some modern dance that is mostly barefoot or multiple disciplines of dance (ie, jazz, hip hop, tap), that may allow us to guide her to a more appropriate type of dance. The male ballet dancer must be able to stand on his forefoot but not en pointe. In addition, he is required to do lifts and carries that are not required of the females.

Once the demographic of this particular patient is determined, the next important thing is to get a history. From a young age, professional dancers are dancing 11 to 12 months a year. It is important to determine exactly when the problem began and the specific symptoms. For this patient, most commonly the symptoms are described as fullness and pain in the posteromedial ankle after a long period of dance. More specifically, the dancer will complain of symptoms when rehearsing and doing a performance. Often there is a change in the dance surface or in the dance intensity that can precipitate the symptoms. Early on, she will almost always ignore and/or dance through the pain with self-administered local ice and oral anti-inflammatories. It is important to determine how much of this self-administered treatment she is receiving in order to truly determine the severity of the symptoms. The perception that the involved ankle has less motion than the contralateral ankle can add to the story. Most often the pain is chronic in nature, and rarely is there an acute episode. By the time professional dancers seek medical care, they have already tried a number of things, including wrapping their ankles and rest.

It is important at this time to understand the specifics of the anatomy in the posterior ankle (Figure 26-1). I often like to describe the posterior ankle as a sandwich waiting to happen. The tibia, talus, and calcaneus are stacked on each other in a very small space. If the talus has either a congenital potentially loose posterior extension, which is termed an *os trigonum*, or a fixed posterior extension, often called the *stieda process*, this posterior extension can get crushed between the tibia and the calcaneus in an athlete who spends most of his or her day in and out of forced plantarflexion. There are also key thickened soft tissue structures that can cause symptoms; specifically, the posterior talofibular ligament and the posterior tibiofibular ligament. This "posterior impingement" is not just a bony impingement but can often be a soft tissue impingement that can present with variants. The first variant in the soft tissue impingement is more of a posterolateral impingement. These patients will complain of posterolateral pain, which is most often a soft tissue impingement, and then a posterocentral and posteromedial pain, which again can be a soft tissue variant of this. Finally, the anatomy of the FHL in the back of the ankle is important to note. The FHL runs directly on the os trigonum or the posterior aspect of the talus on the medial aspect of that structure. The posterior talus is the deep lateral portion to the groove and tunnel that the FHL runs in. Most often, if there is posterior impingement, there is also FHL tendinitis because the 2 structures run so closely together. In addition, an isolated FHL tendinitis can masquerade as a posterior impingement, again because of the anatomic relationship. The FHL runs in a very tight sheath and can get a tenovaginitis in that tendon sheath. The medial position of the FHL is the reason that the symptoms are most often medial.

Physical Examination

The directed physical examination is extremely important and straightforward. There are 2 specific tests that are important in these patients. First, a forced plantarflexion test.

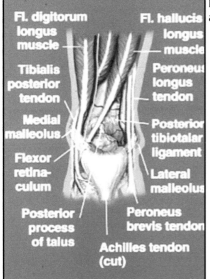

Figure 26-1. Schematic of the anatomy of the posterior ankle.

This is done with the patient's leg bent while the examiner actively plantarflexes the ankle. If there is a significant posterior impingement lesion, this will elicit symptoms consistent with the patient's problem. In addition, asymmetric plantarflexion range of motion can be seen if the plantarflexion test is done bilaterally. The second specific test is a direct palpation on the FHL. Anatomically, this is just behind the neurovascular bundle. Often these patients will be misdiagnosed with Achilles tendinitis because the pain is more posterior than anterior. Once the area of maximum tenderness is palpated medially, it is easy to follow the FHL anteriorly underneath the sustentaculum tali. Most often, in a tendinitis situation, the tenderness goes all the way out. It is very rare to elicit FHL tendinitis symptoms with fixed dorsiflexion of the big toe, so this test is rarely helpful.

Radiographic Evaluation

The radiographic evaluation of these patients is fairly straightforward. In the office, it is very easy to get 3 views of the ankle, and most often any type of bony impingement lesions such as the large stieda process or an os trigonum can be seen quite readily. In addition, it can be helpful for illustrative purposes to get a full plantarflexion x-ray in the office. This often will show the mechanism of the posterior impingement, and it can be instructive to the patient to see that relationship radiographically. Magnetic resonance imaging (MRI) can also be helpful because it allows us to evaluate the FHL tendon itself. The MRI can show if the FHL has attritional tears that may have some prognostic indicators in the treatment of this condition. Edema in the os trigonum or the posterior talar process can also be seen.

Treatment

The initial treatment options should be conservative. Most of these patients, regardless of their level of dance, will get better with a course of physical therapy and rest. The difficulty is getting a professional ballet dancer to rest. If you can get the dancer to take 6 weeks off with a course of physical therapy, friction massage to the FHL, as well as various modalities in that area, the results are good and certainly will keep the dancer off the stage for a shorter period of time than surgery. At the same time, I almost always will have the patient spend some time with her favorite ballet master. A private lesson with a skilled instructor will often illuminate flaws with the dancer's technique that have been longstanding and often may have caused the problem in the first place. All of this can be done during that 6-week period.

The surgical treatment is divided into open and arthroscopic. The open treatment is an incision just posterior to the neurovascular bundle. The neurovascular bundle is exposed. It is important to retract the neurovascular bundle posteriorly and not anteriorly. If you retract it anteriorly, it will require the resection of the medial calcaneal branches, and the patient may now have a better ankle, but also a numb heel. Once the neurovascular bundle is retracted posteriorly, the FHL sheath can be opened easily. It should be released all the way throughout its entire length. At that time a tenosynovectomy plus/minus repair of a tear can be done. Once that is completed, the FHL can be retracted, again posteriorly exposing the posterior aspect of the ankle. The os trigonum and/or prominent talar stieda process can be seen and resected. If the os trigonum is loose and removed easily, it is important to be able to plantarflex fully and have your small finger not be crushed. If it continues to be a problem, then a portion of the posterior talus should be resected with an osteotome or burr. An intraoperative x-ray should be done to make sure that the decompression is complete before closing.

The arthroscopic treatment is one that I have made almost routine in my practice in the last 5 years. Dr. van Dijk from the Netherlands has reported his series of prone posterior arthroscopic ankle and subtalar decompressions for posterior impingement, and my experience has been similar.[2] The portals for the prone arthroscopy are to the medial and lateral side of the Achilles tendon at the level of the tip of the fibula. This operation for an os trigonum is an extra-articular arthroscopic operation. I will use a 4.0 scope with a 4.0 shaver to perform this surgery. It is much more like a shoulder scope than traditional anterior ankle arthroscopy. Once the back of the ankle is exposed, the os trigonum is clearly seen. If it is loose, it can be removed with minimal difficulty with the working portal being the medial side. Of note, all of the work should be kept lateral to the FHL as the neurovascular bundle sits directly medial to the FHL. Once the os trigonum is removed, the FHL sheath is easily exposed. I use a small shaver to débride the sheath. It is important to go at least 1 cm down the sheath to get a complete release of the tendon. At the same time, it is quite easy to do a tenosynovectomy of the involved tendon with a shaver. If there is a tear, I most often will débride the tear with no repair necessary.

The results for this procedure in professional dancers have been excellent. The largest series is Bill Hamilton's out of New York, in which he got his professionals back to full dance over 95% of the time.[1] His results were not as good in amateurs, and this is more than anything, in my opinion, the difficulty with the open treatment. The rehabilitation and resultant scar tissue from the surgery requires a very intense focus for the patient.

My results with arthroscopic treatment have seen a quicker return to dance for even the most casual dancer. It is now the standard in my practice.[3]

The 22-year-old professional ballet dancer is a challenging but rewarding athlete to treat. Most often this condition can be treated conservatively, but open or arthroscopic treatment is certainly easily defended if needed. In my hands, the arthroscopic treatment is superior in results and ease of rehabilitation.

References

1. Hamilton WG, Geppert MJ, Thompson FM. Pain in the posterior aspect of the ankle in dancers. Differential diagnosis and operative treatment. *J Bone Joint Surg Am*. 1996;78(10):1491-1500.
2. van Dijk CN, Scholten PE, Krips R. A 2-portal endoscopic approach for diagnosis and treatment of posterior ankle pathology. *Arthroscopy*. 2000;16(8):871-876.
3. van Dijk CN. Hindfoot endoscopy for posterior ankle pain. *Instr Course Lect*. 2006;55:545-554.

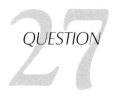
HOW WOULD YOU TREAT A 32-YEAR-OLD TRIATHLETE WITH A NONDISPLACED NAVICULAR STRESS FRACTURE?

Alex J. Kline, MD and Robert B. Anderson, MD

The management of navicular stress fractures in the athlete remains one of the more challenging problems that we face as orthopedic foot and ankle surgeons. Specifically, the decision of whether to operate and the timing of surgical intervention not only require our expertise as surgeons but also must take into account the specific goals of the injured athlete. Prior to determining the best course of action for managing a navicular stress fracture, the diagnosis must first be established. This requires a high index of suspicion in the athlete who develops the insidious onset of dorsal midfoot pain, often described as "ankle" pain. In high-level athletes, the onus is on us to prove or disprove the presence of a stress fracture in a patient who presents with this clinical scenario. If questioned, the athlete may report a recent change in his or her training habits. This is frequently the case in distance runners who are ramping up training for an upcoming race. Initially, these athletes will complain of a vague, aching pain along their dorsal arch that is made worse with the offending activity and relieved with rest. As the condition persists, the pain may become more localized to the dorsal aspect of the navicular.

As a first diagnostic step, a detailed examination of the foot and ankle should be undertaken and the area of maximal tenderness should be determined. If present for some time, tenderness is often elicited at the "N spot" on the dorsal aspect of the navicular. The area of tenderness is often very focal and there is seldom significant swelling noted. Initial imaging should include weight-bearing anteroposterior and lateral radiographs of the symptomatic foot. These should be carefully inspected for the presence of a fracture line, dorsal spur, or reactive sclerosis of the bone. However, it should be noted that initial plain radiographs will be negative in up to 75% of cases, particularly if the fracture is nondisplaced (Figure 27-1). In the athlete with symptoms consistent with a navicular stress fracture and in whom radiographs are normal, further imaging studies are necessary. Bone scans are 100% sensitive in the diagnosis, but they impart little in

Figure 27-1. Anteroposterior radiograph of the foot in a patient with a nondisplaced navicular fracture seen subsequently on a computed tomography (CT) scan.

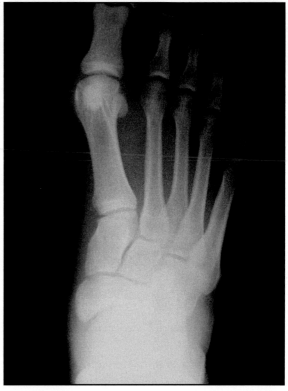

terms of determining the optimal treatment or identifying a true fracture line. Magnetic resonance imaging (MRI) is also sensitive and can perhaps better delineate the extent and location of bone edema (Figure 27-2). However, it will often fail to show a fracture line and is not useful to determine healing. Both MRI and bone scans can be used to confirm the diagnosis, but in terms of helping with my treatment algorithm, a computed tomography (CT) scan gives me the most bang for my buck. The CT scan will show if a fracture line is present, its specific location, and how far it propagates (Figure 27-3).

In a high-level triathlete with a nondisplaced navicular fracture, my first objective would be to learn more about this specific athlete's goals and objectives. Additionally, I would request both an MRI and CT scan to fully assess to what extent the fracture propagates. If the CT scan only identifies a break in the dorsal cortex of the navicular with no propagation of a fracture line or if the MRI shows edema within the navicular and no fracture line on CT scan, I can fairly reliably get this to heal with nonoperative management. However, a strict nonweight-bearing protocol must be employed for at least 6 weeks, and the athlete may not get back to full impact training and participation for 4 to 6 months or more. If the athlete is in an off-season or is willing to undergo this aggressive nonoperative management with prolonged nonweight-bearing, then this is the algorithm that I pursue. In patients in whom the symptoms have been present for several months, I consider augmenting the management with a bone stimulator.

On the other hand, if the CT scan shows that a fracture line extends into the body or extends from the dorsal cortex to a second cortex, I will generally recommend operative management to the patient. The same is true for those showing evidence for propagating

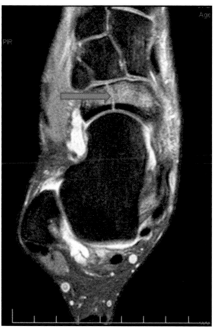

Figure 27-2. T2-weighted axial MRI scan showing edema throughout the navicular with a complete fracture line evident. Arrow shows fracture line.

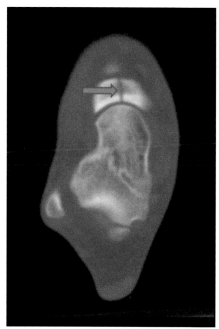

Figure 27-3. Axial CT scan showing complete propagation of a fracture line through both cortices. Arrow shows fracture line.

incomplete fractures on serial CT scans. I find that these fractures heal less reliably even with prolonged immobilization. I review all of these scenarios with the patient, and allow him or her to make an educated decision based on his or her specific needs. In my practice, I find that most high-level athletes want to get back to training faster, and operative intervention provides an opportunity for earlier rehab. It also provides a predictable result; therefore, most will opt for operative management in this scenario.

My algorithm for surgical management of the incomplete or nondisplaced navicular stress fracture is percutaneous screw fixation. If imaging studies show any degree of displacement, or if this is a chronic injury and the imaging studies show sclerosis suggestive of a nonunion, then I will open the fracture and use autologous bone grafting as well. I generally use either calcaneal or distal tibial bone graft for this application. I use 2 4.0-mm partially threaded cannulated screws, inserted perpendicular to the fracture line and usually in a lateral to medial direction (Figure 27-4). Care is taken not to breech the medial cortex, as screw threads may irritate the anterior or posterior tibial tendon (Figure 27-5). It is imperative to have C-arm guidance intraoperatively. In general, I do not advise removing the screws because there is a fairly significant incidence of refracture following screw removal. Postoperatively, I place the patient in a nonweight-bearing cast or boot for 6 weeks, followed by protected weight bearing in a boot with an arch support for another 6 weeks. Then I allow progressive weight bearing and activities as tolerated. We will typically obtain a CT to confirm union prior to letting the athlete return to full competition.

I tend to be fairly aggressive in recommending the operative management of navicular stress fractures. In the incomplete fracture, in which the fracture line does not

Figure 27-4. Intraoperative fluoroscopic image showing placement of the guide pins for 2 cannulated screws.

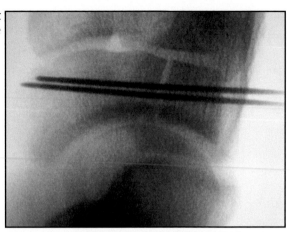

Figure 27-5. Postoperative (A) anteroposterior and (B) lateral radiographs showing placement of 2 cannulated screws.

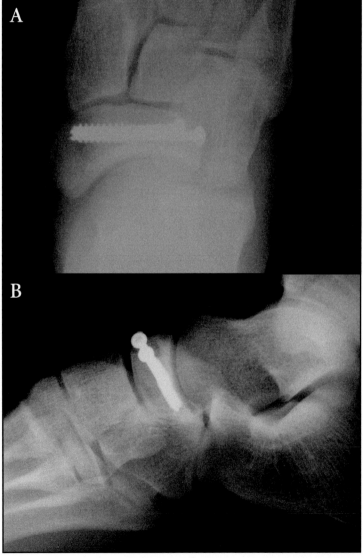

propagate into the body of the navicular, I will attempt nonoperative management if the athlete understands the risks and is willing to go that route following serial CT studies. In any patient with a worsening fracture line or one extending into the body or to another cortex, I feel much more comfortable in percutaneously fixing these fractures with 2 cannulated screws. In my hands, this algorithm works well, and this would be my recommendation to the athlete in this case.

Suggested Readings

Burne SG, Mahoney CM, Forster BB, Koehle MS, Taunton JE, Khan KM. Tarsal navicular stress injury: long-term outcome and clinicoradiological correlation using both computed tomography and magnetic resonance imaging. *Am J Sports Med*. 2005;33(12):1875-1881.

Clanton TO. Is there any question how navicular fractures should be treated? Paper presented at: American Academy of Orthopaedic Surgeons (AAOS) 2009 Annual Meeting. AOFAS/AOSSM Joint Session Specialty Day. February 25-28, 2009; Las Vegas, NV.

Jones MH, Amendonla AS. Navicular stress fractures. *Clin Sports Med*. 2006;25(1):151-158.

Lee S, Anderson RB. Stress fractures of the tarsal navicular. *Foot Ankle Clin*. 2004;9(1):85-104.

Potter NJ, Brukner PD, Makdissi M, Crossley K, Kiss ZS, Bradshaw C. Navicular stress fractures: outcomes of surgical and conservative management. *Br J Sports Med*. 2006;40(8):692-695.

Saxena A, Fullem B. Navicular stress fractures: a prospective study on athletes. *Foot Ankle Int*. 2006;27(11):917-921.

MY 25-YEAR-OLD PATIENT IN WHOM I HAVE PREVIOUSLY PLACED A JONES SCREW FOR A FIFTH METATARSAL STRESS FRACTURE NOW HAS NEW PAIN WITH A POSITIVE TRIPLE PHASE BONE SCAN. NOW HOW DO I TREAT THIS PATIENT?

Bruce Cohen, MD

To begin a discussion of the treatment of fifth metatarsal fractures, it is important to clarify the definition and describe the fracture types. The fifth metatarsal fracture was initially described in 1902 by Dr. Robert Jones. This fracture was noted to have a significant risk of nonunion that was described as high as 20%. These fractures are classified based on zones of vascular anatomy, fracture location, and chronicity.[1,2]

Fractures of the fifth metatarsal have been divided into 3 zones. Zone I is described as the tuberosity fractures with primarily cancellous bone and a relatively low risk of nonunion or functional problems. Zone II fractures are located at the metaphyseal/diaphyseal junction of the fifth metatarsal and the fracture line enters into the articulation between the bases of the fourth and fifth metatarsals. Zone III fractures are distal to the fourth/fifth intermetatarsal ligament and extend distally into the tubular portion of the diaphysis. The Zone II fractures are commonly referred to as "Jones fractures" and the Zone III fractures are typically stress fractures. The clinical importance of this differentiation is the healing rates of these fractures, which is related to the vascular anatomy. The Zone I fractures have a superior healing rate to the more distal fractures.[3,4]

The fracture is differentiated as either acute or a stress fracture by the location of the fracture as well as the presence of intramedullary sclerosis. Sclerosis of the intramedullary canal indicates chronicity of the fracture. When a fracture is identified to have intramedullary sclerosis, this is typically treated with intramedullary fixation as well as concomitant bone grafting.[4]

When a fifth metatarsal is treated operatively, intramedullary fixation is the fixation of choice. We prefer to use a solid screw inserted through an incision proximal to the metatarsal base. The screw diameter is chosen based on the fit noted intraoperatively. The largest screw that reasonably fits is chosen. In patients with long-standing intramedullary sclerosis, the screw diameter chosen is frequently smaller than the typical acute fracture. When deciding on thread length, the threads should just cross the fracture site. It is important to avoid placing a longer screw due to the subtle curvature of the bone in the distal half.

Complications from the operative treatment of fifth metatarsal fractures have been reported as high as 45%. These complications are most frequently related to technical issues. The insertion site of the screw is critical and I emphasize the "high and inside" location. As the osteology of the fifth metatarsal demonstrates a distal curvature, distal bone penetration can occur when using a screw that is too long or poor insertion location is used. With these technical errors, nonunion or delayed union may occur. A bent or broken screw is indicative of a nonunion. Other complications include peroneal tendonitis from a prominent screw head and sural nerve injury (usually iatrogenic).

Continued pain after fixation of a fifth metatarsal fracture is most frequently the result of a delayed union or nonunion. In the treatment of these fractures, it is critical to follow the healing radiographically. This is typically done with standard radiographs but can be confirmed with computed tomography scans. Another factor that may contribute to failure of operative treatment is mechanical overload from hindfoot varus.

In the case of the patient with recurrence of pain after fixation of a fifth metatarsal fracture, there are many factors to consider. The first factor is whether the fracture truly united after fixation. This needs to be carefully examined on radiographs. Details to note are the presence of bridging bone and cortical hypertrophy. Of course the screw needs to be examined closely to look for deformation or failure. An excessively long screw may cause pain distally due to cortical encroachment. An improper insertion site of the screw will cause possible medial cortex penetration if started too laterally. The second factor to discuss is the overall foot position. Excessive hindfoot varus will cause lateral column overload and may lead to recurrent fractures or nonunion.

In the presence of a positive bone scan with what was felt to be a previously healed fracture, the initial treatment would be conservative, including rest, possible immobilization, and activity limitation. In a competitive athlete, the length of time of activity limitation will depend on the timing of the season and competition. If the radiographs demonstrate no new fracture lines or evidence of hardware malposition, attention must be made to location and size of the implant. If there is any early evidence of hardware failure or refracture, then I would recommend revision surgery with a larger diameter solid implant. If there is a fracture line or cleft, then open bone grafting or the use of biologics is recommended. I prefer the use of calcaneal bone graft for small areas or iliac crest for significant nonunions with significant intramedullary sclerosis (Figures 28-1 and 28-2).

If the pain persists after failure of an appropriate period of conservative care, then surgical intervention must be seriously considered. Very careful examination of standing alignment is likely to demonstrate a hindfoot varus with pes cavus. If this is present, along with revision fixation of the metatarsal, a valgus-producing calcaneal osteotomy and/or a dorsiflexion osteotomy of the first metatarsal should be performed (Figure 28-3).

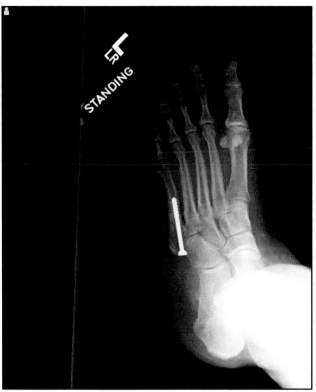

Figure 28-1. Anteroposterior radiograph postfixation of Jones fracture.

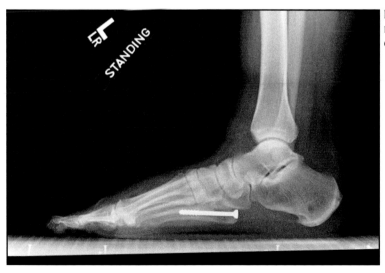

Figure 28-2. Lateral radiograph postfixation of Jones fracture.

Adjuvant treatments should also be considered. The use of bone stimulation with ultrasound or electromagnetic techniques can be used in this situation. There is no definitive evidence of efficacy in the use of nonunions of the fifth metatarsal, but it can be used in the high-level athlete. The use of appropriate orthotic devices is very important postoperatively as these patients get back to activity and athletic competition. This will typically consist of an orthotic with lateral posting as well as a turf toe plate or lateral ray

Figure 28-3. Lateral radiograph post valgus-producing osteotomy.

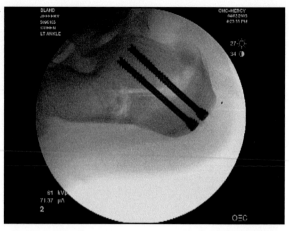

rigid extension. The length of time to return to sport is somewhat variable depending on the presence or absence of radiographic union. Computed tomography confirmation of solid osseous union is recommended prior to return to active competition.

The final comment is to leave the screw in place following surgery regardless of primary or revision surgery. The refracture risk is significant following screw removal, especially in an athlete.

Conclusion

There are many factors to consider when evaluating the painful fifth metatarsal following fixation. Implant size, location, and evidence of failure must be carefully evaluated. Continued pain despite appropriate conservative treatment typically requires revision fixation with consideration of adjuvant bone grafting or biologic stimulation. Careful attention to foot alignment is critical. Hindfoot or forefoot realignment osteotomy can be used to correct hindfoot varus or first ray plantarflexion.

References

1. Jones R. Fractures of the base of the fifth metatarsal bone by indirect violence. *Ann Surg.* 1902;35(6):697-700.
2. Dameron TB Jr. Fractures and anatomical variations of the proximal portion of the fifth metatarsal. *J Bone Joint Surg.* 1975;57(6):788-792.
3. DeLee JC, Evans JP, Julian J. Stress fractures of the fifth metatarsal. *Am J Sports Med.* 1983;11(5):349-353.
4. Torg JS, Balduini FC, Zelko RR, Pavlov H, Peff TC, Das M. Fractures of the base of the fifth metatarsal distal to the tuberosity. *J Bone Joint Surg.* 1984;66(2):209-214.

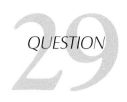
How Do You Treat a 21-Year-Old Basketball Player Who Has Magnetic Resonance Imaging Evidence of Tibial Diaphyseal Edema Not Resolved After 3 Months of Protected Weight Bearing?

Jeremy A. Alland, BA and Shane J. Nho, MD, MS

The patient is a 21-year-old male basketball player who originally presented with magnetic resonance imaging (MRI) evidence of tibial diaphyseal edema. The edema is unresolved after 3 months of protected weight bearing. It is suspected that the patient is experiencing a stress fracture of the tibia.

The tibia is the most common site for a stress fracture, representing as much as 75% of the total occurrence in certain patient populations. A study in 2005 reported Finnish military recruits as a high-risk population for stress fractures, appearing in as much as 64% of the population.[1] The general athletic population has a relatively low incidence (<1%), but the subpopulation of runners has an incidence of approximately 20%.[1] The vast majority appear as transverse fractures; however, longitudinal fractures do occur.

Risk factors can be caused by genetic abnormalities or can be developed through overuse. Congenital and developmental factors, such as smaller tibial width and knee malalignment, have been shown to be associated with stress fractures.

Tibial stress fractures are classified as either low risk or high risk based mostly upon the specific location of the injury. Low-risk fractures appear on the posterior medial tibia, representing an injury due to compression. A low-risk injury is unlikely to progress to complete failure. High-risk fractures are less common and appear in the middle third of the anterior cortex, representing an injury to the tension aspect of the tibia. High-risk injuries often progress to complete failure and result in significant further injury if untreated.[2]

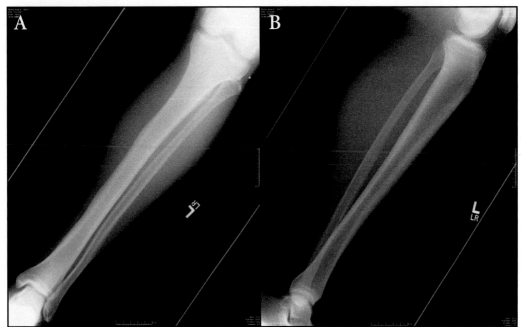

Figure 29-1. Plain radiographs of left tibia for a 22-year-old runner with distal tibial pain. (A) Anteroposterior view without evidence of fracture. (B) Lateral view without evidence of fracture.

The physician should first take a detailed history of the patient to aid in the differential diagnosis. It is important to discuss how long the patient has been symptomatic and to get a description of the pain. Determine the intensity of the pain, the location, what makes it worse, and what makes it better. Also discuss the patient's daily athletic activity, both before and after the injury. Additionally, the patient's dietary habits and supplements are also important information to obtain. For female patients, the female triad of anorexia, amenorrhea, and osteoporosis should be considered in any stress fracture.

After a sufficient history, the physician should conduct the physical exam. The physician should palpate the leg, buttocks, and lower back as the injury permits. The range of motion and strength of the limb must be examined. Also of importance is the gait of the patient; pay close attention to any compensation or abnormalities. The physician should check the distal circulation, sensation, and mobility, and stretch the patient's toes to elicit associated pain. Lastly, laboratory tests should be obtained to determine if there is evidence of infection, blood clot, or tumor based on clinical suspicion. If the patient has had recurrent stress fractures, the physician should obtain a dual-emission X-ray absorptiometry scan and basic laboratory serum calcium, albumin, 25-hydroxyvitamin D, phosphorus, and bone alkaline phosphatase. More extensive workup should warrant a referral to a metabolic bone specialist.

A physical exam that indicates a possible stress fracture must be imaged to provide a complete differential diagnosis. In the office setting, orthogonal views using plain radiographs of the tibia can be obtained at the initial presentation (Figure 29-1). It can take over a month after the onset of pain to be reflected in a plain radiograph, and therefore, may not be diagnostic for acute injuries.[3] MRI is the most effective diagnostic tool for the tibial stress fracture (Figure 29-2).

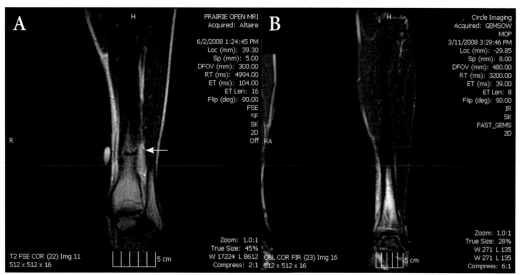

Figure 29-2. MRI images. (A) Coronal T2-weighted image demonstrating a stress fracture at the anterior aspect of the middle tibia. (B) Sagittal T2-weighted image demonstrating increased signal in the middle aspect of the anterior tibia. (Arrow) Stress fracture.

A bone scan may also be used to confirm the diagnosis. A stress fracture shows fusiform uptake, which differs from the linear uptake of shin splints.

This patient has MRI evidence of tibial diaphyseal edema that is unresolved with 3 months of protected weight bearing. Due to the unresolved edema, shin splints can be ruled out, which should resolve with protected weight bearing. Periostitis would also resolve with protected weight bearing. The laboratory tests can provide some indication if infection, blood clot, or tumor is a potential cause of the injury. Basketball does not generally restrict the blood flow to the tibial region, which rules out exercise-induced compartment syndrome. The diagnosis is most likely tibial stress fracture. Basketball players spend a considerable amount of time jumping, which would place the patient at risk of compression side injury. A compression injury occurs at the posterior medial tibia and is considered low risk.

A low-risk tibial stress fracture rarely proceeds to complete fracture, and therefore, the treatment remains conservative with nonsurgical options. Initial treatment involves restriction of all activity to prevent weight bearing. The physician may recommend a pneumatic leg brace, which decreases force and increases venous congestion at the area of the injury.[4] The patient will be prescribed analgesia with the dosage based upon weight and age. If the injury prevents proper gait, crutches can be prescribed. Other noninvasive treatment options (ie, bone stimulator, pulsed ultrasound) have not shown to improve healing from rest and weight-bearing restrictions.[5,6] Low-risk fractures generally heal in 1 to 2 months, with return to play in 3 to 4 months. The symptoms, however, tend to improve in 2 to 6 weeks, and the patient may gradually return to activities when the edema and pain are resolved.

In the case of a high-risk stress fracture of the anterior tibia (tension injury), the athlete cannot return to play until the fracture is completely healed. The treatment of a high-risk injury should initially follow the same conservative options as the low-risk injury.

For high-risk fractures, it usually requires 4 to 6 months to completely resolve with rest and immobilization, at which point, the patient can gradually return to play. If the conservative approach is not effective, a surgical approach may be considered. An intramedullary nailing of the tibia in cases of stress fractures has been shown to be effective in patients that were unresponsive to a minimum of 4 months of nonoperative management.[7] Radiographic healing of the fracture postoperation occurs after approximately 3 months and return to play occurs around 4 months. Surgical complications include anterior knee pain and recurrence of the fracture. Intramedullary nailing has been shown to be more effective than external fixation in terms of tibial alignment, but there are no differences in infection rates and healing time.[8]

The 21-year-old patient may gradually return to activities with resolution of symptoms and after 2 to 6 weeks of immobilization, analgesics, and rest. If pain and swelling remain, the immobilization should be continued for a full 1 to 2 months. Without pain and swelling, the patient may return to play in approximately 3 to 4 months. The physician may indicate a return to play earlier with complete resolution of the symptoms and imaging indications. The patient should be monitored for circulation issues due to the pneumatic brace. Surgical options should be avoided for this patient if possible.

References

1. Valimaki V, Alfthan H, Lehmuskallio E, et al. Risk factors for clinical stress fractures in male military recruits: a prospective cohort study. *Bone.* 2005;37(2):267-273.
2. Kaeding CC, Yu JR, Wright R, Amendola A, Spindler KP. Management and return to play of stress fractures. *Clin J Sport Med.* 2005;15(6):442-447.
3. Heyworth BE, Green DW. Lower extremity stress fractures in pediatric and adolescent athletes. *Curr Opin Pediatr.* 2008;20(1):58-61.
4. Swenson EJ, DeHaven KE, Sebastianelli WJ, Hanks G, Kalenak A, Lynch JM. The effect of a pneumatic leg brace on return to play in athletes with tibial stress fractures. *Am J Sports Med.* 1997;25(3):322-328.
5. Beck BR, Matheson GO, Bergman G, et al. Do capacitively coupled electric fields accelerate tibial stress fracture healing? *Am J Sports Med.* 2008;37(3):545-553.
6. Rue JP, Armstrong DW, Frassica FJ, Deafenbaugh M, Wilckens JH. The effect of pulsed ultrasound in the treatment of tibial stress fractures. *Orthopedics.* 2004;27(11):1192-1195.
7. Varner KE, Younas SA, Lintner DM, Marymount JV. Chronic anterior midtibial stress fractures in athletes treated with reamed intramedullary nailing. *Am J Sports Med.* 2005;33(7):1071-1076.
8. Henley MB, Chapman JR, Agel J, Harvey EJ, Whorton AM, Swiontkowski MF. Treatment of type II, IIIA, and IIIB open fractures of the tibial shaft: a prospective comparison of unreamed interlocking intramedullary nails and half-pin external fixators. *J Orthop Trauma.* 1998;12(1):1-7.

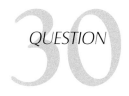

How Do You Treat "Shin Splints" in the High-Level Athlete Who Needs to Continue to Compete?

Jeremy A. Alland, BA and Shane J. Nho, MD, MS

A high-level athlete reports to your clinic with pain around the anterior tibia. The athlete participates in intense exercise a minimum of 5 days a week. It is suspected that the athlete is experiencing a form of medial tibial stress syndrome (MTSS) and needs to return to play as soon as possible.

MTSS, more commonly referred to as shin splints, is one of the most common lower leg injuries in sports. Certain studies have reported 6% to 16% of all injuries in a running population as a form of MTSS.[1] The incidence is higher in populations that often participate in running, jumping, and sprinting.

MTSS is a form of periostitis as a result of excessive stress on the medial border of the tibia, primarily involving the soleus but also the flexor digitorum longus and the deep crural fascia.[2,3] The proposed mechanism of injury occurs when there is excessive strain on the soleus from foot hyperpronation or the velocity of pronation with repetitive impact activities, increase in the duration or intensity of activities, or changes in training surface.[4] There are a number of proposed risk factors, which makes prevention incredibly difficult. MTSS can arise from gait abnormalities, such as increased foot pronation, increased muscular strength of the plantarflexors, soft tissue injuries such as muscular tightness or insertional anomalies, or increased varus tendency of the forefoot or hindfoot. More commonly, acute changes in exercise regiments cause the onset of MTSS, including abrupt increases in training intensity or duration, hard or inclined running surfaces, and inadequate equipment.

Patients generally complain of dull, achy pain located in the distal aspect of the posteromedial tibia. The pain is generally worse with activity and impairs performance but relieves with rest. Determine the patient's daily athletic regiment, both before and after the injury, as MTSS typically occurs after a change in intensity, frequency, or duration of training. Additionally, the patient's dietary habits and supplements are also important information to obtain. For female patients, the female triad of anorexia, amenorrhea, and osteoporosis in stress reactions should be considered.

The physical examination begins with observation of the gait as well as evidence of excessive hindfoot alignment, particularly valgus and/or forefoot hyperpronation. In MTSS, patients will have vague pain with tenderness to palpation over the posteromedial tibia from the middle to distal third. There may be occasional associated soft tissue swelling. The area of pain is more generalized in MTSS rather than the point tenderness associated with tibial stress fractures. Some patients may have pain with toe raises or resisted plantarflexion.[4] The range of motion and strength of the limb must be examined. The physician should check the distal circulation, sensation, and mobility, and stretch the patient's toes to elicit associated pain. Lastly, laboratory tests should be obtained to determine if there is evidence of infection, blood clot, or tumor based on the clinical exam. Because MTSS may present similar to posterior tibial tendonitis in presentation and examination, careful physical exam to the region of pain is vital.

Diagnostic workup for MTSS begins with plain radiographs. Radiographs are usually normal, but there can be evidence of cortical hypertrophy with diffuse periosteal new bone formation.[4] Magnetic resonance imaging is not a reliable study for MTSS, but it is useful for ruling out stress fractures, tumor, and posterior tibial tendon pathology or pathologic lesions of the tibia. A 3-phase bone scan demonstrates longitudinal lesions of the posteromedial cortex in MTSS as opposed to more focal uptake in stress fractures.

The case describes a high-level athlete with intense and frequent training that likely contributed to the onset of MTSS. Rest is the most important treatment for MTSS and may take up to 4 months. The athlete should avoid all activity for a short period of time. Ice may be beneficial in the early presentation as well as nonsteroidal anti-inflammatory medications (NSAIDs). If the patient has evidence of hindfoot or forefoot deformities, the patient should be fitted for appropriate orthotics or running shoes. The athlete may initiate a pain-free, nonimpact, cross-training program (swimming or cycling) to maintain aerobic fitness with a gradual return to training intensity or duration and running surfaces. For many patients, the combination of activity modification and NSAIDs will be enough to increase healing and allow for return to play in a short period of time.

For cases that do not respond to initial conservative treatment and activity modification, a pneumatic boot has been shown to decrease force and increase venous congestion around the tibia, both of which encourage healing.[5] Surgery is rarely advocated for patients with MTSS.

The athlete diagnosed with MTSS may return to play as soon as all pain and swelling are resolved. Any recurrence of the injury must be reported immediately and treated in order to prevent more serious injury. After the athlete returns to play, it is important to focus on the prevention of future injury. A previous incident with MTSS is a significant risk factor for a future recurrence. There are a few preventive measures that can be taken for the athlete. A weak or fatigued muscle cannot absorb force as well as a healthy, rested muscle. Shock-absorbent insoles, as well as regular replacement of athletic shoe wear, dissipate shock and prevent the force from reaching bone, which decreases the occurrence of tibial stress injuries.[1] Another important preventive tactic is the use of graduated running programs, more absorptive surfaces, and preseason conditioning. As mentioned previously, abrupt changes in training intensity has been a proposed risk factor for tibial stress injuries. Therefore, reducing the distance, intensity, and frequency of training sessions at the beginning of the season can reduce chances of injury.[1]

References

1. Craig DI. Medial tibial stress syndrome: evidence-based prevention. *J Athl Train.* 2008;43(3):316-318.
2. Beck BR, Osternig LR. Medial tibial stress syndrome: the location of muscles in the leg in relation to symptoms. *J Bone Joint Surg Am.* 1994;76:1057-1061.
3. Beck BR, Matheson GO, Bergman G, et al. Do capacitively coupled electric fields accelerate tibial stress fracture healing? *Am J Sports Med.* 2008;37(3):545-553.
4. Pell RF IV, Khanuja HS, Cooley GR. Leg pain in the running athlete. *J Am Acad Orthop Surg.* 2004;12(6):396-404.
5. Swenson, EJ, DeHaven KE, Sebastianelli WJ, Hanks G, Kalenak A, Lynch JM. The effect of a pneumatic leg brace on return to play in athletes with tibial stress fractures. *Am J Sports Med.* 1997;25(3):322-328.

What Is Your Technique for an Achilles Tendon Repair? What Is Your Cut-Off for a Primary Repair and How Do You Treat Them if Greater Than That?

Christopher P. Chiodo, MD

The question of when is it "too late" to proceed with the primary repair of an acute Achilles tendon rupture is based on several factors. Further, generalizations are difficult and the decision to proceed with surgery in patients presenting beyond 2 weeks from the time of injury must be made on a case-by-case basis.

In active individuals in whom there has been a delay in diagnosis and in whom there is a palpable gap in the tendon, it is never "too late." These patients should undergo primary repair with mobilization of the proximal segment and the use of a V-Y advancement and/or flexor hallucis longus tendon transfer if necessary. Alternatively, in a less active individual who presents 3 to 4 weeks out from the time of injury, and in whom there is no palpable gap present, surgery may not be necessary.

Other factors to consider in the decision-making process include the condition of the skin envelope, comorbidities (diabetes, vascular disease, dermatological conditions), and anticipated patient compliance.

If it is decided to proceed with surgery, I prefer the use of an open repair modified from that technique reported by Mandelbaum and colleagues.[1,2] The salient features of the technique include a medial longitudinal incision, a nonstrangulating Krackow stitch, a posterior compartment fasciotomy, no tourniquet, a layered closure (including the paratenon), and aggressive perioperative antibiotics.

The patient is positioned prone on the operating table under general, spinal, or regional anesthesia. The extremity is prepped in the standard fashion using a bristled alcohol scrub followed by povidone-iodine paint.[3] A well-padded thigh tourniquet is applied but not inflated. Avoiding the use of a tourniquet is important for 2 reasons. First, it allows continuous tissue and flap perfusion. Second, and probably more importantly, it ensures

Figure 31-1. Posteromedial incision. (Copyright © 2010 by the American Orthopaedic Foot and Ankle Society, Inc., originally published in *Foot & Ankle International*, 2008;29(1):114-118 and reproduced here with permission.)

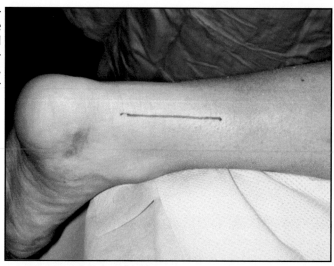

Figure 31-2. Paratenon incision. (Copyright © 2010 by the American Orthopaedic Foot and Ankle Society, Inc., originally published in *Foot & Ankle International*, 2008;29(1):114-118 and reproduced here with permission.)

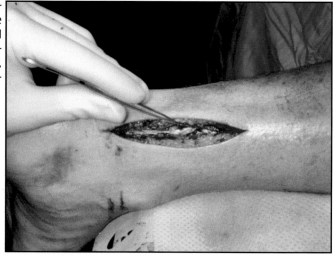

meticulous hemostasis throughout the case and therefore minimizes the chance of hematoma formation (and subsequent dehiscence).

A 12- to 15-cm medial longitudinal skin incision is used (Figure 31-1). I never use a lateral or central incision as these can result in sural nerve injury or scar irritation from the shoe counter. Sharp dissection is carried straight down to the paratenon, which is then isolated just enough such that a distinct layer is visible for closure at the end of the case. The paratenon is then incised longitudinally in line with the skin incision (Figure 31-2). Great care is taken not to delaminate the subcutaneous adipose from the skin and not to mobilize deep flaps until the paratenon has been incised.

The tendon rupture is identified and mobilized. If present, the "mop ends" are not débrided. The main reason for this is to maintain tendon length. Overaggressive tendon débridement and resection can lead to a gap that necessitates a repair with the ankle in excessive equinus. This, in turn, may predispose to re-rupture.

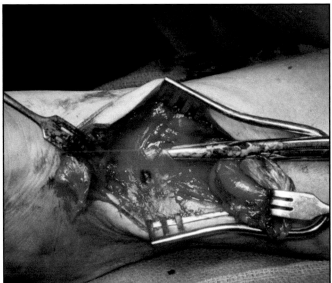

Figure 31-3. Posterior compartment fasciotomy. (Copyright © 2010 by the American Orthopaedic Foot and Ankle Society, Inc., originally published in *Foot & Ankle International*, 2008;29(1):114-118 and reproduced here with permission.)

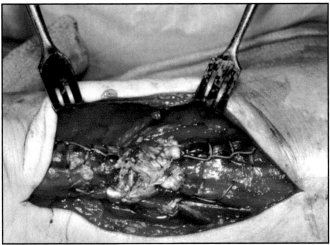

Figure 31-4. Repair using a Krackow stitch. (Copyright © 2010 by the American Orthopaedic Foot and Ankle Society, Inc., originally published in *Foot & Ankle International*, 2008;29(1):114-118 and reproduced here with permission.)

Next, a posterior compartment fasciotomy is performed, slightly lateral to the midline and extending the length of the repair (Figure 31-3). This step increases the space available to accommodate any postoperative tissue edema and drainage. More importantly, it facilitates a complete closure of the paratenon at the end of the case, especially if there is a bulky tendon repair.

The tendon repair is then performed. I use a locked, nonstrangulating Krackow stitch,[4] usually with #2 Ethibond suture (Ethicon, Somerville, NJ; Figure 31-4). This technique is biomechanically superior to the Bunnell and Kessler repairs.[5] A 2-stranded repair is usually sufficient, and the sutures should enter the tendon anteriorly such that the knots are away from the skin. If necessary, the repair may be augmented with a #1 or 0 Vicryl suture (Ethicon), taking care not to violate the primary suture line.

With regard to the tension of the repair, the goal should be physiologic resting ankle equinus. This is usually about 10 degrees. The contralateral extremity is a helpful guide

Figure 31-5. Paratenon closure. (Copyright © 2010 by the American Orthopaedic Foot and Ankle Society, Inc., originally published in *Foot & Ankle International*, 2008;29(1):114-118 and reproduced here with permission.)

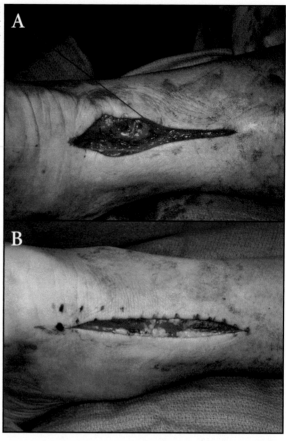

and for this reason may be sometimes prepped draped into the operative field. If there is excessive tension on the repair, it will be manifested by excessive ankle equinus. To minimize this, the proximal tendon segment should be mobilized prior to tying the sutures. To do so, axial traction is held on this segment with the sutures in place but not tied. While doing so, adhesions between the gastrocnemius muscle and its fascia are manually broken up with a long finger or blunt malleable retractor. If there is still excessive equinus after performing this maneuver, I do not hesitate to add gastrocnemius recession or even V-Y lengthening to the procedure.

Once the tendon repair is complete, attention is turned toward closure. This is a critical step of the procedure as wound problems have been a historic concern in Achilles tendon repair.[6] I am always able to close 3 layers. The first is the paratenon, which is closed with a running 0 or 2-0 Vicryl suture (Figure 31-5). For me, this is one of the most critical steps of the procedure, as it protects the repair and also takes tension off of the skin and subcutaneous closure. Again, the previous posterior fasciotomy substantially facilitates this step of the procedure. After the paratenon, the subcutaneous tissues are closed with buried 4-0 Monocryl sutures (Ethicon). I prefer Monocryl to Vicryl as I find that Monocryl evokes less tissue reaction and attendant "spitting" of the stitch. Finally, 3-0 or 4-0 nylon sutures are used to close the skin using a no-touch technique.

Postoperatively, patients are immobilized for 10 to 14 days in a nonweight-bearing posterior splint with the ankle in approximately 10 degrees of equinus. Thereafter, they begin home range-of-motion exercises, specifically active dorsiflexion and gravity plantarflexion for 5 minutes 3 times per day. I now allow patients to be partial weight bearing in a boot at 2 weeks postoperatively, incorporating a heel lift that ranges from 1 to 3 inches, based on the tension of the repair. This is reduced by half at 4 weeks postoperatively. By 6 weeks postoperatively, the patient is permitted full weight bearing in a boot with a 1/4" to 3/8" lift. The boot is discontinued between 9 and 12 weeks postoperatively. I had previously kept patients completely nonweight bearing for 6 weeks, but this changed in light of a recent investigation demonstrating improved outcomes with early weight bearing.[7] Finally, most patients are now anticoagulated for 4 weeks postoperatively. The reason for this is that we had a 4% incidence of venous thromboembolic disease in our 100-patient series.[8]

In recent years, the question of whether a minimally invasive repair should be considered arises. In one recent trial comparing this technique to an open repair, the outcomes were similar while complications were lower in the minimally invasive group.[9] Nevertheless, using the open technique described presently, we have found no wound complications (including infections), no nerve injuries, and only one instance of a partial re-rupture in a large consecutive series.[8]

References

1. Mandelbaum BR, Myerson MS, Forster R. Achilles tendon ruptures. A new method of repair, early range of motion, and functional rehabilitation. *Am J Sports Med.* 1995;23(4):392-395.
2. Chiodo CP, Den Hartog B. Surgical strategies: acute Achilles rupture-open repair. *Foot Ankle Int.* 2008;29(1):114-118.
3. Keblish DJ, Zurakowski D, Wilson MG, Chiodo CP. Preoperative skin preparation of the foot and ankle: bristles and alcohol are better. *J Bone Joint Surg Am.* 2005;87(5):986-992.
4. Krackow KA, Thomas SC, Jones LC. A new stitch for ligament-tendon fixation. Brief note. *J Bone Joint Surg Am.* 1986;68(5):764-766.
5. Watson TW, Jurist KA, Yang KH, Shen KL. The strength of Achilles tendon repair: an in vitro study of the biomechanical behavior in human cadaver tendons. *Foot Ankle Int.* 1995;16(4):191-195.
6. Wills CA, Washburn S, Caiozzo V, Prietto CA. Achilles tendon rupture. A review of the literature comparing surgical versus nonsurgical treatment. *Clin Orthop Relat Res.* 1986;(207):156-163.
7. Suchak AA, Bostick GP, Beaupré LA, Durand DC, Jomha NM. The influence of early weight-bearing compared with non-weight-bearing after surgical repair of the Achilles tendon. *J Bone Joint Surg Am.* 2008;90(9):1876-1883.
8. Petty C, Duggal N, DeAsla R, Chiodo CP. Minimizing peri-operative complications associated with open repair of acute Achilles tendon rupture: the results of a prospective, multi-center protocol. Paper presented at: Annual Summer Meeting of the American Orthopedic Foot and Ankle Society; July 16, 2009; Vancouver, British Columbia, Canada.
9. Aktas S, Kocaoglu B. Open versus minimal invasive repair with Achillon device. *Foot Ankle Int.* 2009;30(5):391-397.

How Do You Treat an Athlete With Chronic Lateral Foot Overload and Peroneal Tendonitis With a Cavovarus Foot?

Brian C. Toolan, MD

My approach to an athlete with a symptomatic cavovarus foot begins with characterizing the deformity and appreciating how it contributes to pedal dysfunction. In my experience, without a thorough understanding of the derivation of a cavovarus deformity and an effective plan to correct each of its constituent malalignments, successful and lasting resolution of the manifestations secondary to the cavovarus foot will not occur, even with appropriate treatment of the associated manifestations.[1]

A Coleman block test is my first step in determining if the varus heel associated with the cavovarus foot is arising from the hindfoot or whether it is being "driven" by a deformity in the forefoot (Figure 32-1). Positioning the affected foot with the first metatarsal lying off the edge of the 1-inch high block allows the first ray to drop off and eliminates the contribution of any fixed forefoot valgus deformity to the alignment of the heel. If the heel corrects out of varus during this test, 2 characteristics of the cavovarus foot have been determined. First, a forefoot valgus deformity due to plantarflexion of the first metatarsal is present, and it is driving the heel into a compensatory varus position. Second, this hindfoot deformity is flexible and the subtalar joint is mobile. If the heel does not change position when the first ray drops off the edge of the block, then a fixed varus deformity is present in the hindfoot. Under these circumstances, failure to address the hindfoot directly will not resolve the varus heel. Thus, even if the forefoot is realigned properly, the patient will continue to experience difficulties with pedal function.

My evaluation to identify the etiology of painful, chronic lateral overload in a cavovarus foot begins with a careful physical exam with the patient in the lateral decubitus position. I palpate the fifth metatarsal and look for callosities underneath its head, shaft, and base and along the lateral border of the foot. Bony tenderness and swelling suggest the possibility of an acute fracture, a stress injury, or a chronic nonunion. A malunion with dorsiflexion of the metatarsal can be appreciated. I check for swelling behind the

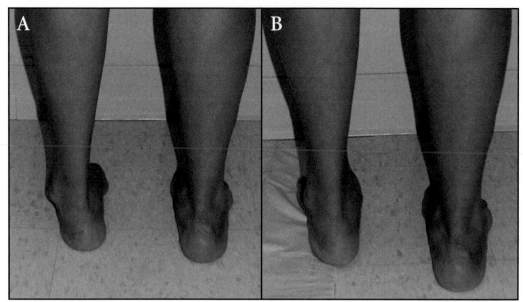

Figure 32-1. Evaluation of a varus heel in a patient with a cavovarus foot deformity. (A) A 15-degree varus alignment of the heel. (B) The hindfoot deformity is flexible because the heel corrects into valgus during a Coleman Block test.

lateral malleolus and along the lateral border of the foot. I palpate along the course of the eroneal tendons during active eversion. As I assess the strength of eversion, I observe whether the peroneal tendons subluxate during active contraction. With the patient in this position, it is easier to distinguish eversion of the foot from plantarflexion of the first ray, so I can better assess the integrity of the brevis and longus tendons. Lastly, I inspect the alignment of the entire limb to ensure that there is no deformity of the ankle, knee, or hip that could be contributing to the foot malalignment. Weight-bearing anteroposterior, lateral, and oblique views of the foot may reveal a fracture, bony changes due to prior injury, and joint pathology. Magnetic resonance imaging (MRI) may be requested to confirm suspicious radiographic findings. I prefer MRI for its capacity to provide comprehensive and specific visualization of bony, articular, and soft-tissue anatomy of the foot and ankle.

My treatment of lateral foot overload depends on the results of my workup and the duration of symptoms. Acute conditions are defined as those with an onset of 4 to 6 weeks without a prior history of similar complaints. This would include first-time, acute fracture; stress or trauma; a stress reaction of the bone; peroneal tendonitis; and a painful os peroneum. I render conventional treatment for these conditions and prescribe physical therapy and corrective foot orthosis to address the flexible cavovarus deformity. These patients perform eversion strengthening, proprioceptive training, and wear orthosis with a first ray drop-off and lateral heel posting. If a painful os peroneum demonstrates migration proximal to the calcaneocuboid joint on an oblique radiograph of the foot suggesting significant tearing or complete rupture of the peroneus longus tendon, I perform surgery to excise this sesamoid and tenodese the longus to the brevis. Chronic conditions include recurring or persistent conditions lasting more than 3 months. Nonunions of the fifth metatarsal, lateral process of the talus, anterior process of the calcaneus, tearing or

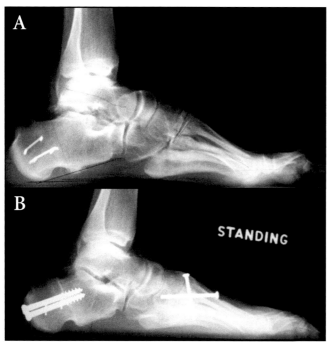

Figure 32-2. Weight-bearing lateral radiographs of a 26-year-old male with persistent lateral foot pain and tendinitis of the peroneus brevis despite undergoing a calcaneal osteotomy during his adolescence. (A) The preoperative radiograph demonstrates a plantarflexed first metatarsal that is causing the varus alignment of the heel to persist. (B) Postoperative radiographs obtained 1 year after a dorsiflexion arthrodesis of the first tarsometatarsal joint, transfer of the peroneus longus to brevis to strengthen eversion of the foot, and a revision calcaneal osteotomy to further translate the tuber into valgus

instability of the peroneal tendons, and lateral ligamentous instability warrant consideration of surgical management with simultaneous correction of the cavovarus deformity.[2] For a cavovarus foot deformity that is driven by a plantarflexed first ray, a dorsiflexion osteotomy at the base of the first metatarsal is indicated. A lateral displacement osteotomy of the calcaneal tuberosity is necessary when the Coleman block test does not demonstrate correction of the varus position of the hindfoot with elimination of the effect of a forefoot valgus. A hindfoot fixed in varus with arthritis of the subtalar joint may be treated with an arthrodesis to reduce pain and achieve a valgus heel. Often, releases and tendon transfers are combined with these bony procedures to balance the soft tissues. The plantar fascia may be partially or completely released, the posterior tibial and Achilles tendon lengthened, and the peroneus longus transferred to the peroneus brevis in order to realign the cavovarus foot into a plantigrade position (Figure 32-2).

Most patients, including my athletes, are skeptical of the contribution of their cavovarus foot to their presenting complaints. They often rationalize that if their foot has been "crooked" since birth, why didn't it cause a problem before? Although some remain unconvinced, a review of their past history of injuries; difficulties with activities on uneven surface inclines; and their balance during pivoting, jumping, and cutting combined with an explanation of a cavovarus foot with an anatomical model frequently persuades them to accept the treatment plan. Often, true acceptance comes when they appreciate the decrease in their overall level of discomfort and the subtle difficulties with their feet along with the resolution of their presenting complaint. The most satisfied patients are those who finally attain relief of chronic, nagging problems that had eluded them for several years despite numerous physician visits, physical therapy sessions, orthotics, and operations that had failed to yield improvement in their function.

References

1. Manoli A, Graham B. The subtle cavus foot, "the underpronator." *Foot Ankle Intl.* 2005;26(11):256-263.
2. Younger ASE, Hansen ST. Adult cavovarus foot. *J Am Acad Orthop Surg.* 2005;13:302-315.

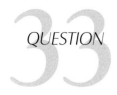

How Do You Manage a
Significant Turf Toe Injury?

Nicholas R. Seibert, MD and Robert B. Anderson, MD

Injuries to the hallux metatarsophalangeal (MTP) joint are not uncommon, particularly in the running athlete.[1-7] One of the more common mechanisms of hallux injury is a hyperextension force on a foot fixed to the ground in equinus. The subsequent ligamentous injury has been termed *turf toe*.[2] The incidence of this injury has been on the rise and is thought to be the result of shoe/cleat-surface interaction, especially among football players on artificial turf.[6] The severity of this injury can range from a mild sprain to frank dorsal dislocation of the hallux. Assessing the location and extent of soft tissue damage as well as any associated bony abnormalities is the first step in determining treatment and expected outcome.

Clinical exam exhibits swelling and tenderness about the hallux MTP joint. Ecchymosis of the plantar surface is often present. The resting position of the hallux should be noted and compared to the contralateral, uninjured foot to determine any malalignment. Loss of active motion is a common finding in the acute phase, but it is important to test the function of both the flexor hallucis brevis (FHB) and the flexor hallucis longus (FHL) during physical exam. Stability of the hallux MTP joint is the most important finding on physical exam. The vertical Lachman test is performed by holding the first metatarsal fixed and translating the hallux dorsally to determine vertical stability. It is also important to check varus and valgus stability, as variants of this injury exist that disrupt the collateral ligaments, particularly the medial structures, which may predispose to the athlete to progressive hallux valgus.[1,7]

Radiographic exam provides the most important information in determining whether operative intervention is warranted. Weight-bearing anteroposterior and lateral views of the forefoot should be obtained; however, they often provide little information by themselves. Fractures of the sesamoid, capsular avulsions, or varus/valgus angulation of the hallux may be evident. Contralateral views are recommended to gauge proximal migration of the sesamoid complex, a sign of complete rupture of the plantar plate (Figure 33-1). Live fluoroscopic evaluation is indispensable in evaluating these injuries. Passive and active motion of the hallux can demonstrate plantar soft tissue disruption by a lack

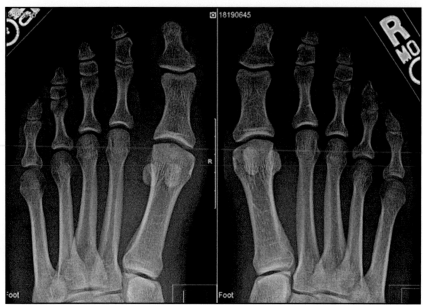

Figure 33-1. Weight-bearing AP foot x-rays demonstrate retraction of the sesamoid complex on the left, when compared to the normal right foot.

of sesamoid excursion. This is not only invaluable diagnostic information, but also provides the patient with education and an understanding of the injury pattern. Magnetic resonance imaging has also become a standard part of the evaluation of these injuries.[8] It provides excellent anatomic detail of the soft tissue, osseous, and articular structures and helps to guide the treatment plan, as well as prognosis and return to play (Figure 33-2).

Initial treatment is similar to most other soft tissue injuries and consists of RICE (rest, ice, compression, elevation). Nonsteroidal anti-inflammatory medications are useful in this phase of healing. The foot may be immobilized in a walking boot or cast with a toe spica extension. Taping or bracing can be used to pull the hallux into slight plantarflexion and varus to bring the injured tissues into opposition. Gentle range of motion can often be started several days after injury. Most athletes with low-grade injuries can return to play with taping or a rigid turf toe orthotic, as symptoms allow. Significant turf toe injuries often take several months to fully recover from. It is important to take into account an athlete's sport, position, and specific requirements when deciding on a treatment plan.

Operative treatment of turf toe injuries is seldom required. Indications for surgery include the failure of nonoperative treatment with persistent pain and the inability to push-off or progressive deformity. Surgical intervention in the acute setting may also be considered for the following situations:

1. A large capsular avulsion with unstable joint (especially medial)
2. Diastasis of bipartite sesamoid or sesamoid fracture
3. Retraction of sesamoids (single or both)
4. Traumatic bunion/progressive hallux valgus
5. Positive (+) vertical Lachman test
6. Loose body or chondral injury

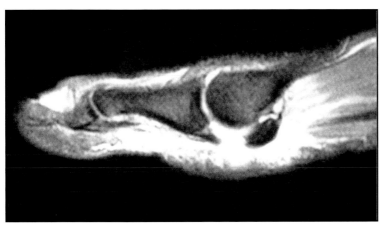

Figure 33-2. An MRI demonstrating disruption of the plantar plate with edema and proximal migration of the sesamoid. Note the remaining distal tissue used for surgical repair.

Surgical approaches include a longitudinal plantar medial incision that may be extended along the plantar surface in the flexor crease at the MTP joint or separate medial and plantar incisions. It is our practice to use separate incisions because it allows better wound healing and improved visualization of the lateral FHB complex. It is important to identify and protect the plantar digital nerves during the approach. Always evaluate the FHL tendon for split tears. The goal of surgery is primary anatomic repair of the injured tissues. This proceeds from lateral to medial and often can be performed with nonabsorbable suture, as a cuff of tissue is typically present at the base of the proximal phalanx. If the distal soft tissues are inadequate, suture anchors or drill holes may be required to secure the repair to the phalanx.

If a medial injury exists and a traumatic bunion had developed, a "modified McBride" bunionectomy can be performed in conjunction with the soft tissue repair. This removes the valgus deforming force of the adductor hallucis tendon. If there is diastasis or fracture of a sesamoid, we prefer to excise the smaller pole and repair the remaining soft tissue defect. Internal fixation of a sesamoid fracture proves to be a humbling experience. If the entire sesamoid must be excised, transfer of the abductor hallucis tendon may be considered. This not only provides tissue to fill the defect, but also functions as a dynamic flexor of the joint. Late reconstruction of these injuries is more difficult and may require lengthening of tissues proximal to the sesamoids or an FHL recession transfer for cock-up deformity of the hallux.

Postoperative rehabilitation strikes a delicate balance between soft tissue healing and early mobilization. Initially the hallux should be wrapped into slight plantarflexion and varus and the leg immobilized in a splint. Gentle passive range of motion and active plantarflexion under supervision can begin 7 to 10 days after surgery. The patient should remain nonweight bearing in a removable splint or boot for 4 weeks. Removable bunion splints can be used to protect the repair, especially at night. At 4 weeks, weight bearing in a boot is allowed. Transition to normal shoe wear with an appropriate turf toe plate or orthotic is allowed at 8 weeks. High-level athletes can expect return to sport at 3 to 4 months but may not see full recovery for 6 to 12 months.

References

1. Anderson RB. Turf toe injuries of the hallux metatarsophalangeal joint. *Tech Foot Ankle Surg*. 2002;1(2):102-111.
2. Bowers KD Jr, Martin RB. Turf-toe: a shoe-surface related football injury. *Med Sci Sports*. 1976;8(2):81-83.
3. Clanton TO, Ford JJ. Turf toe injury. *Clin Sports Med*. 1994;13(4):731-741.
4. Clanton TO, Butler JE, Eggert A. Injuries to the metatarsophalangeal joints in athletes. *Foot Ankle*. 1986;7(3):162-176.
5. Coker TP, Arnold JA, Weber DL. Traumatic lesions of the metatarsophalangeal joint of the great toe in athletes. *Am J Sports Med*. 1978;6(6):326-334.
6. Rodeo SA, O'Brien S, Warren RF, et al. Turf-toe: an analysis of metatarsophalangeal joint sprains in professional football players. *Am J Sports Med*. 1990;18(3):280-285.
7. Watson TS, Anderson RB, Davis WH. Periarticular injuries to the hallux metatarsophalangeal joint in athletes. *Foot Ankle Clin*. 2000;5(3):687-713.
8. Tewes DP, Fischer DA, Fritts HM, et al. MRI findings of acute turf toe. A case report and review of anatomy. *Clin Orthop Relat Res*. 1994;304:200-203.

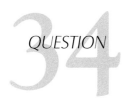
HOW LONG DO HIGH ANKLE SPRAINS REALLY TAKE TO GET BETTER? HOW DO YOU EVALUATE THEM APPROPRIATELY?

Jennifer Chu, MD and Judith Baumhauer, MD, MPH

High ankle sprain is a term used to describe injury to the syndesmotic ligaments. They consist of the anteroinferior tibiofibular ligament, posteroinferior tibiofibular ligament, interosseous ligament, inferior transverse ligament, and interosseous membrane. In addition to direct palpation for tenderness over the syndesmosis, your physical examination should include the squeeze test and the external rotation test. The squeeze test involves compressing the fibula against the tibia above the mid-calf level. If the syndesmosis is injured, this will cause the bones to separate distally and the patient will feel pain at the syndesmosis. The external rotation test is positive when externally rotating the foot with the leg stabilized and the knee flexed to 90 degrees results in pain at the syndesmosis.[1,2] The external rotation test can also be performed under fluoroscopy to look for disruption of the normal symmetrical ankle mortise relationship.

You should obtain weight-bearing anteroposterior, lateral, and mortise views of the ankle. Ankle radiographs should be examined for widening of the medial clear space between the talus and medial malleolus as well as widening of the tibiofibular clear space between the medial fibula and incisura fibularis. Suspect syndesmotic injury if the medial clear space on the mortise view is greater than 4 mm or greater than the distance between the tibial plafond and superior talar dome.[2] Injury should also be suspected if the tibiofibular clear space measured 1 cm above the tibial plafond is greater than 6 mm on anteroposterior or mortise x-rays, or if the tibiofibular overlap 1 cm above the tibial plafond is less than 1 mm on a mortise view or less than 6 mm on an anteroposterior view (Figure 34-1). You should also consider radiographs of the tibia and fibula to evaluate for a Maisonneuve injury, an interosseous ligament injury that exits through the proximal fibula.

Stress views of the ankle will allow you to determine the stability of a syndesmotic injury. If the syndesmosis is unstable, externally rotating the foot relative to the leg should

Figure 34-1. The tibiofibular clear space (indicated by the open arrows) should measure <6 mm in both the anteriorposterior and mortise views. The tibiofibular overlap (solid arrows) should measure <6 mm on the anteroposterior view and less than 1 mm on the mortise view. (Reprinted with permission from Katcherian D. Soft-tissue injuries of the ankle. In: Lutter LD, Mizel MS, Pfeffer GB, eds. *Orthopaedic Knowledge Update: Foot and Ankle.* Rosemont, IL: American Academy of Orthopaedic Surgeons; 1994:241-253.)

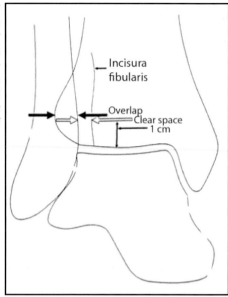

Figure 34-2. External rotation stress view of a Weber B distal fibula fracture. Widening of the medial clear space >4 mm on the mortise view indicates a syndesmotic injury.

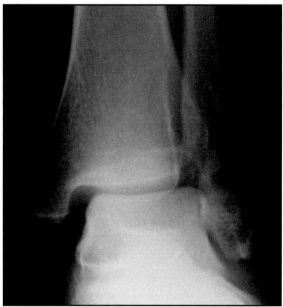

result in widening of the medial clear space on a mortise view (Figure 34-2) and posterior translation of the fibula relative to the incisura fibularis on lateral view.

Healing time for stable high ankle sprains is variable and dependent on the rehabilitation protocol.[1] Studies in athletes show that time missed from sports can be up to 7 to 8 weeks, which is twice as long as for ankle sprains without injury to the syndesmotic ligaments. Treatment principles for stable high ankle sprains are the same as for inversion ankle sprains: rest, ice, compression, and elevation. For patients with significant pain or poor muscle activation, complete immobilization and compression through a cast or splint should be considered. An ankle brace may be considered for patients without

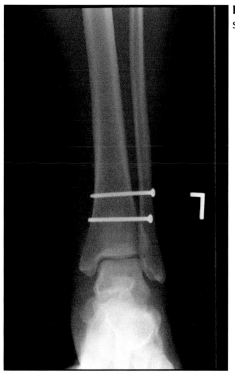

Figure 34-3. Placement of 2 bicortical syndesmotic screws.

significant pain. You should determine the level of weight bearing immediately after the injury based on the patient's pain and the severity of the injury. I place patients in a removable walking boot and allow progressive weight bearing as tolerated. I begin physical therapy immediately to decrease swelling and encourage range of motion. I have patients wear the boot for up to 3 weeks and transition them to an ankle brace when they are walking without a limp and the swelling has nearly subsided. Progressive functional ankle rehabilitation exercises are then implemented under a physical therapist's guidance 2 times a week for 6 weeks.

Unstable syndesmotic injuries, where widening of the medial clear space or tibiofibular clear space is seen either on initial or stress radiographs, should be treated with reduction and transsyndesmotic fixation (Figure 34-3). Current controversies regarding transsyndesmotic fixation include whether metallic or bioabsorbable screws should be used, whether 1 or 2 screws should be used, whether a suture-button ("tightrope") device should be used, whether 3 or 4 cortices should be drilled prior to screw placement, and whether metallic screws should be removed. The available literature does not clearly answer any of these questions.[1,3] My practice is to use 2 metal screws, drill 3 cortices 1 cm above the distal tibiofibular joint, and insert screws with the ankle in dorsiflexion. I do not routinely remove screws, but I do tell patients that screw breakage is likely to occur with return to activity. Following surgery, I will keep patients nonweight bearing for 6 to 8 weeks but do allow ankle motion in a removable boot. After this period, I allow patients to begin progressive weight bearing in a removable boot and then progress them to an ankle brace. I tell my patients that they will usually not be able to return to sports until at least 8 to 12 weeks after their injury.

References

1. Williams G, Jones M, Amendola A. Syndesmotic ankle sprains in athletes. *Am J Sports Med.* 2007;35(7):1197-1207.
2. Zalavras C, Thordarson D. Ankle syndesmotic injury. *J Am Acad Orthop Surg.* 2007;15(6):330-339.
3. Aronow M, Sullivan R. Ankle sprains and ligament injuries. In: DiGiovanni C, Greisberg J, eds. *Foot and Ankle: Core Knowledge in Orthopaedics.* Philadelphia, PA: Elsevier/Mosby; 2007:235-237.

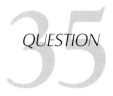

How Do You Treat Chronic Ankle Instability in Your Recreational Athletes?

Johnny Lin, MD and Nickolas G. Garbis, MD

Evaluation and treatment of chronic ankle instability in the recreational athlete can often be a frustrating situation. Feelings of chronic ankle instability can be persistent in up to 20% of patients who have sustained acute inversion sprains to the ankle.[1] A course of physical therapy focused on peroneal strengthening and proprioception may help improve symptoms, but a certain percentage of these patients will continue to have instability. In general, a high-level athlete is more likely to be managed surgically when dealing with chronic ankle instability, whereas a more sedentary person may be better suited with a course of physical therapy and appropriate rehabilitation of the secondary stabilizers in the ankle, along with activity modification and bracing. The recreational athlete falls in the middle of these 2 groups, as most of them do want to return to sport and are not willing to avoid the activities that cause their symptoms of instability.

History and Physical Exam

The diagnosis of chronic ankle instability begins with a thorough history. Many of these patients will present with complaints of recurrent inversion sprains, pain, and difficulty walking on uneven ground. When they come to the office for evaluation, it is important to get an accurate picture of when they are symptomatic and what sort of treatment they have already received. I try to get a sense of whether the ankle impedes them in their activities of daily living or if it is mostly bothersome with sports. It is also important to ask patients if they are using any sort of bracing for their ankle and if they feel it helps their symptoms. On physical examination, it is important to first observe the alignment of the hindfoot as varus alignment can predispose a patient to recurrent ankle sprains and can lead to failure of operative treatment if it is not addressed. The ankle joint itself should be examined for any crepitation or pain with range of motion. The joint line should be palpated medially and laterally. Pain along the joint line may signify a concomitant osteochondral lesion. The anterior talofibular ligament (ATFL) and

Figure 35-1. The anterior drawer test is done with the ankle in a slight amount of plantarflexion. The "suction" sign is seen and is considered an abnormal finding.

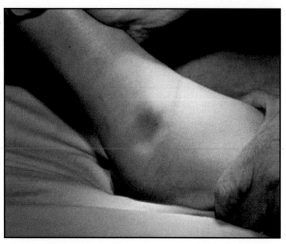

calcaneofibular ligament (CFL) should be palpated for tenderness or edema. The course of the peroneal tendons should be palpated for any tenderness or crepitation to identify secondary peroneal tendon pathology. Chronic dislocation of the peroneal tendons can also be identified with resisted eversion from a plantarflexed and inverted position. Eversion strength should be tested, as inappropriately rehabilitated peroneal tendons will not be able to act as secondary stabilizers in the chronically unstable ankle. When examining the ankle for laxity, it is important to compare it to the contralateral side. I like to test the ATFL with the foot in slight plantarflexion (Figure 35-1). I usually place my thumb on the lateral malleolus with my fingers wrapping around the back of the foot. Since the deltoid ligament complex is intact, it is usually easier to detect laxity by performing a rotatory motion as opposed to a pure anterior drawer. When evaluating the CFL, I like to keep the foot in neutral dorsiflexion, grasp the hindfoot with the thumb on the lateral process of the talus and the fingers on the medial hindfoot, and invert the ankle. The amount of laxity is compared to the opposite side.

Diagnostic Testing

Diagnostic imaging is also important in characterizing the pathology of the ankle. I will start by obtaining 3 standard weight-bearing radiographs of the ankle. Any osteochondral lesions or peroneal tendon pathology may be further evaluated with magnetic resonance imaging if clinically suspected. In addition, any signs of joint degeneration such as joint space narrowing or osteophytes should be noted. I routinely get standardized stress views of the ankles to measure talar tilt and anterior translation of the talus. This is done with a Telos Stress Device (Metax GmbH, Hungen, Germany) using 20 N of force. When measuring anterior translation, I measure from the talus (Figure 35-2) to the posterior edge of the plafond. In accordance with the literature, I consider the presence of instability with anterior drawer testing with an absolute value of 9 mm, or 5 mm greater than the normal side. When measuring talar tilt on a mortise stress radiograph, an absolute angle >10 degrees or an angle 5 degrees greater than the normal side between the articular surfaces of tibia and talus is indicative of laxity (Figure 35-3).[2]

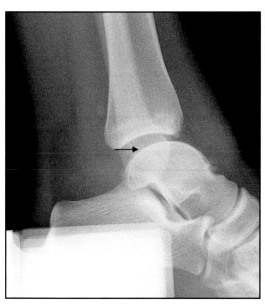

Figure 35-2. Stress lateral radiograph illustrating an abnormal anterior drawer. The arrow demonstrates how the distance is measured between the posterior tibia and the talus.

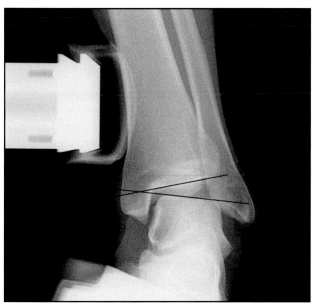

Figure 35-3. Stress mortise radiograph illustrating an abnormal talar tilt test. The talar tilt angle is shown by measuring the angle between the articular surface of the tibia and talus.

Management

When making the determination for surgery, most patients should try an initial course of nonoperative management. This includes physical therapy for functional exercises and peroneal strengthening and the use of an off-the-shelf ankle brace. Lace-up braces are usually more effective than taping and elastic sleeves; however, I frequently employ taping and bracing together during sporting activities. Most recreational athletes will be satisfied with rehab and functional bracing.[3] A small percentage of patients will continue to have symptoms of ankle instability. In recalcitrant cases, operative reconstruction is offered.

Figure 35-4. Intraoperative photo showing repair of the lateral ligaments using suture anchors. Sutures are shown grasping the ligaments. The superior border of the lateral extensor retinaculum is shown being held by the tissue forceps.

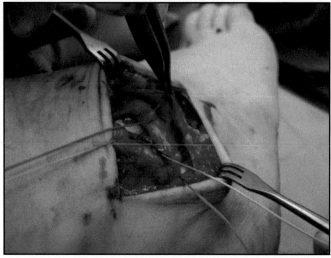

When discussing operative management with the patient, most of the time my preference is to perform the Broström procedure with the Gould modification. This procedure is considered an anatomic repair of the lateral ligaments. Both the ATFL and the CFL are exposed. Frequently there is no clear rupture of the ligaments, but they are attenuated and elongated. When elongated, the redundant ligament is excised and repaired back to the fibula either through drill holes or suture anchors (Figure 35-4). In addition, the Gould modification is added to reinforce the repair using the superior border of the lateral extensor retinaculum, which is seen distal to the ATFL and CFL in Figure 35-4. There are also several tenodesis procedures that have been described to treat chronic lateral instability. While tenodesis and augmented repairs tend to be stronger, they also limit subtalar motion and can significantly alter hindfoot biomechanics so they are not a first line of treatment in my practice. Anatomic reconstruction can be expected to be successful in greater than 80% of patients.[4] In revision cases or in those patients who exhibit generalized ligamentous laxity, I use either an autograft or allograft hamstring tendon to anatomically reconstruct the ATFL and CFL. I prefer the use of interference screws to fix the graft into the talus, fibula, and calcaneus.[5] Bony deformity is addressed if there is an underlying varus deformity of the hindfoot with a Dwyer lateral closing wedge calcaneal osteotomy. A parallel incision posterior and inferior to the original incision for the Broström ligament repair is chosen, taking care to maximize the skin bridge.[6] The typical postoperative protocol involves splinting the ankle in slight eversion and neutral plantarflexion and maintaining nonweight bearing for 2 weeks. This is followed by a 2-week period of weight bearing in a short leg cast. At 4 weeks postoperatively, a removable cast boot is placed and physical therapy is begun for range-of-motion and strength exercises. The cast boot can be transitioned into an off-the-shelf lace-up ankle brace at the 6- to 8-week postoperative visit, and activity can slowly be advanced as tolerated. Full speed sport activities are permitted 3 to 4 months after surgery.

References

1. Freeman MA. Instability of the foot after injuries to the lateral ligament of the ankle. *J Bone Joint Surg Br.* 1965;47(4):669-677.
2. Ahovuo J, Kaartinen E, Slätis P. Diagnostic value of stress radiography in lesions of the lateral ligaments of the ankle. *Acta Radiol.* 1988;29(6):711-714.
3. Malliaropoulos N, Papacostas E, Papalada A, Maffulli N. Acute lateral ankle sprains in track and field athletes: an expanded classification. *Foot Ankle Clin.* 2006;11(3):497-507.
4. Gould N, Seligson D, Gassman J. Early and late repair of lateral ligament of the ankle. *Foot Ankle.* 1980;1(2):84-89.
5. Colville MR. Surgical treatment of the unstable ankle. *J Am Acad Orthop Surg.* 1998;6(6):368-377.
6. Maffulli N, Ferran NA. Management of acute and chronic ankle instability. *J Am Acad Orthop Surg.* 2008;16(10):608-615.

SECTION V

TRAUMA

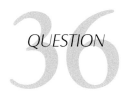

How Do You Treat Proximal Fifth Metatarsal Fractures?

Carroll P. Jones, MD

There are 3 distinct fracture patterns that affect the base of the fifth metatarsal. Unfortunately, the terminology and descriptions of these injuries remain confusing in the orthopedic literature. Diagnostic clarity is critical as it dictates treatment recommendations and prognosis.

Quill[1] reported a classification of fifth metatarsal base fractures based on 3 zones (Figure 36-1). Zone I fractures occur through the tuberosity and are considered avulsion injuries. Zone II fractures are more distal and extra-articular (relative to the tarsometatarsal joint) and traverse the 4-5 intermetatarsal articulation. Fractures in the proximal portion of the diaphysis are considered Zone III. Sir Robert Jones' original description involving 4 cases, including his own, were acute fractures in the Zone II region.[2]

The most common fracture of the fifth metatarsal base is an avulsion of the tuberosity. Although originally thought to be caused by overpull of the peroneus brevis tendon when the foot supinates or adducts abruptly, literature has supported the notion that the lateral band of the plantar fascia is the primary cause.[3] I treat the vast majority of tuberosity fractures in a hard-soled shoe or short Controlled Ankle Movement boot with full weight bearing permitted. The more symptomatic patients with lower pain tolerances typically do better with the walker boot. Patients are encouraged to transition to regular shoes as soon as they feel comfortable, which is usually 3 to 4 weeks after the injury. I do not routinely obtain follow-up radiographs because fibrous unions are common, are usually asymptomatic, and do not change my treatment recommendations.

Occasionally, I will see a patient with a large Zone I tuberosity avulsion that involves a significant amount of the joint surface. If substantial joint displacement is noted (more than 2 to 3 mm), I will consider open reduction and internal fixation. Computed tomography is very helpful in evaluating the extent of the joint involvement and displacement if plain films are equivocal. For these relatively uncommon variants, I use a small fragment screw placed obliquely through the tuberosity and across the medial cortex of the proximal fifth metatarsal in lag fashion. A partially threaded cannulated 4.0-mm screw with a

Figure 36-1. Zones and fracture patterns of the fifth metatarsal base.

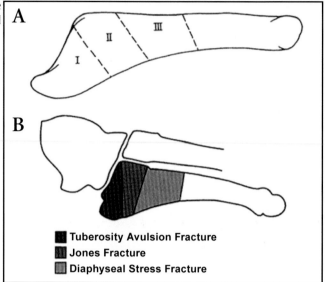

washer works well. I expose the fracture through a longitudinal incision centered on the dorsal aspect of the tuberosity and place the screw percutaneously. Postoperatively, I keep these patients nonweight bearing for the first 2 to 3 weeks in a splint, and then advance to protected weight bearing in a cast or boot until 6 weeks after surgery.

A true Jones fracture is an acute injury that occurs in Zone II of the fifth metatarsal base (Figure 36-2). Treatment for these fractures is controversial. Nonoperative treatment in a nonweight-bearing short leg cast has been the traditional treatment[4] and is still widely practiced. Clapper et al[5] reported average time to healing of 21 weeks and a 28% nonunion rate from a series of 25 patients with a true acute Jones fracture. I favor the use of a walker boot, and permit weight bearing as tolerated in patients who choose to avoid surgery. Anecdotally, we have not appreciated a higher nonunion rate with this approach compared to nonweight bearing in a cast. For most cases, however, I offer operative treatment to the patient. The surgery is relatively simple with low morbidity and it facilitates faster and higher union rates with a more aggressive rehabilitation. Most practitioners recommend surgical intervention in all high-performance athletes, but I apply this to any patient who desires a more reliable, shorter healing period, albeit with the risk of surgery.

For patients electing surgery for an acute Jones fracture, I recommend percutaneous intramedullary screw fixation. The procedure can be performed under an ankle block as an outpatient. A guide-pin is placed under fluoroscopy through a small incision. The starting point is critical to optimize screw placement. A "high and inside" starting location on the base of the fifth metatarsal facilitates maintaining an intramedullary screw position with avoidance of cortical break-out in a bone with curved morphology. I use a cannulated entry system but place a solid, partially threaded screw, usually 4.5 or 5.5 mm in diameter. Ideal screw length is just long enough for the threads to be distal to the fracture (Figure 36-3). Typically, the screw traverses about half of the metatarsal length. I do not routinely bone graft the acute Jones fractures. Postoperatively, patients are nonweight bearing in a splint for 2 weeks, then full weight bearing in a walker boot until 6 to 8 weeks postoperatively. Activity is progressed based on symptoms and radiographic healing. Return to full activity, including sports, may take up to 3 months.

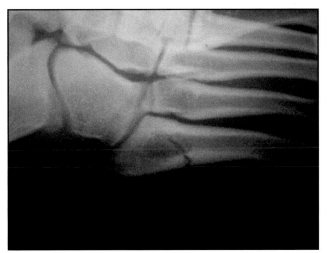

Figure 36-2. Acute Zone II Jones fracture.

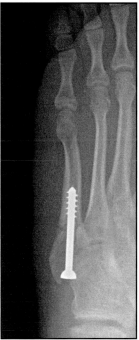

Figure 36-3. Appropriate intramedullary screw position with ideal screw length.

Zone III injuries in the proximal diaphysis of the fifth metatarsal are typically stress fractures (Figure 36-4). Patients often report prodromal symptoms, but radiographic findings are variable. Torg et al have classified these as acute or chronic.[6] Acute fractures are typically characterized by a radiolucent line with sharp margins and minimal bone hypertrophy. Chronic stress fractures, including delayed and nonunions, typically demonstrate a widened lucent line with resorption, intramedullary sclerosis, and periosteal reaction. Acute proximal diaphyseal stress fractures are treated similar to acute Jones fractures, and expectedly are equally controversial. Nonweight bearing in a short leg cast is an accepted treatment, although I will typically allow weight bearing in a walker boot and add the use of an external bone stimulator.

Depending on the patient's preferences and goals, I favor intramedullary screw fixation for acute and chronic Zone III stress fractures. It is critical to assess hindfoot alignment, and varus position is a contributing factor both in terms of etiology and recurrent fractures. I will add a hindfoot osteotomy in severe cases, or if the patient has failed previous screw fixation. The percutaneous technique for screw fixation is the same as noted for Jones fractures. For nonunions and delayed unions, I will also make a small incision over the fracture site and débride the bone and fibrous tissue. The defect is then packed with autograft, usually a small dowel of bone from the calcaneus or iliac crest. Postoperative protocol includes nonweight bearing for 2 weeks in a splint, followed by protected weight bearing in a walker boot until 6 to 8 weeks after surgery. For high-risk cases (ie, revision surgery or nonunions), I also use an external bone stimulator and the rehabilitation process is less aggressive.

Figure 36-4. Zone III diaphyseal acute stress fracture.

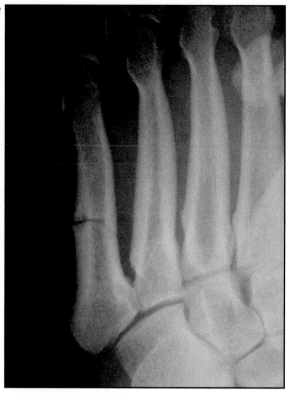

Conclusion

It is critical that any fracture of the fifth metatarsal base is appropriately assessed in terms of both location and chronicity. Prognosis and treatment is vastly different for the many variants, and an understanding of the classification will facilitate appropriate management.

References

1. Quill GE. Fractures of the proximal fifth metatarsal. *Orthop Clin North Am.* 1995;26:353-361.
2. Dameron TB. Fractures and anatomical variations of the proximal portion of the fifth metatarsal. *J Bone Joint Surg Am.* 1975;57:788-792.
3. Richli WR, Rosenthal DI. Avulsion fracture of the fifth metatarsal: experimental study of pathomechanics. *Am J Roentgenol.* 1984;143:889-891.
4. Rosenberg GA, Sferra JJ. Treatment strategies for acute fractures and nonunions of the proximal fifth metatarsal. *J Am Acad Orthop Surg.* 2000;5:332-338.
5. Clapper MF, O'Brien TJ, Lyons PM. Fractures of the fifth metatarsal: analysis of a fracture registry. *Clin Orthop.* 1995;315:238-241.
6. Torg JS, Balduini FC, Zelko RR, Pavlov H, Peff TC, Das M. Fractures of the base of the fifth metatarsal distal to the tuberosity: classification and guidelines for non-surgical and surgical management. *J Bone Joint Surg Am.* 1984;66:209-214.

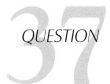

How Do You Manage a 22-Year-Old College Lineman With a Minimally Displaced or Ligamentous Lisfranc Injury?

Terrence M. Philbin, DO and Jaymes D. Granata, MD

Midfoot sprains in athletes are low velocity injuries that can be easily missed or under-appreciated. Although rare in the general population, Lisfranc injuries in athletes occur more often, with the highest incidence in football lineman.[1,2] The classic mechanism of injury in a football player is an indirect injury that occurs with the foot plantarflexed and the metatarsophalangeal joints fixed in maximum dorsiflexion. When a vertical axial load is applied (eg, another player falling onto the heel), the Lisfranc joint complex is injured through hyperplantarflexion. The weaker dorsal capsuloligamentous structures fail first, followed by the interosseous and strong plantar ligaments. This leads to a wide spectrum of injury with often subtle radiographic findings. It is important to have a strong index of suspicion when evaluating a midfoot complaint in an athlete and to investigate the injury beyond apparently normal nonweight-bearing radiographs. In one series, 50% of displaced Lisfranc ligament injuries were missed on initial nonweight-bearing views.[3]

Making the diagnosis of a minimally displaced Lisfranc injury may not always be straightforward. We combine a thorough history and physical exam along with appropriate imaging studies to clarify the extent of injury. Our treatment recommendations are based on whether the injury has resulted in instability across the Lisfranc joint complex. Both stable sprains and unstable ligament tears may present similarly on physical exam. Athletes generally complain of an inability to return to sport due to painful weight bearing. The affected foot is often swollen and tender to palpation. The presence of ecchymosis on the plantar aspect of the foot should raise your suspicion for a significant midfoot injury (Figure 37-1).

Initial imaging studies include 3 weight-bearing views of both feet. On the anteroposterior (AP) view, we look at the alignment of the medial border of the second metatarsal and the medial aspect of the middle cuneiform, the 1-2 intermetatarsal space, as well as any obvious diastasis between the navicular and cuneiform articulations. The oblique

Figure 37-1. Plantar ecchymosis after a Lisfranc joint complex injury.

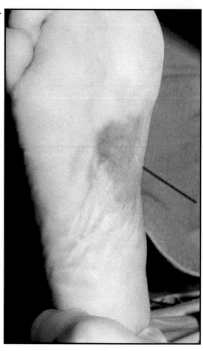

view allows for visualization of the third and fourth tarsometatarsal (TMT) joints. The lateral view may demonstrate dorsal-plantar displacements at the TMT joints. It also shows the relationship between the medial cuneiform and the fifth metatarsal. If the medial cuneiform is plantar to the fifth metatarsal, the arch height has collapsed, indicating an unstable Lisfranc ligament complex injury.

Many of the athletic Lisfranc injuries will involve the first and second TMT articulations. For small displacements of 1 to 5 mm, the only radiographic abnormality may be the 1-2 intermetatarsal distance on the AP weight-bearing view. We recommend using a comparison view of the contralateral foot for a more accurate interpretation of subtle diastasis (Figure 37-2).

If the weight-bearing views do not reveal any displacement or instability, we will order a magnetic resonance imaging (MRI) and consider manual fluoroscopic stress views under anesthesia. MRI can better define the ligamentous injury and obviate the need for an exam under anesthesia in some cases. A recent study found MRI to be accurate in the distinction between stable and unstable Lisfranc ligament injuries in 90% of their cases.[3] We still recommend the use of fluoroscopic stress views under anesthesia in the operating room if the above workup is equivocal, with consent for open reduction and internal fixation if warranted. Stress abduction views may show disruption of the medial column line on true AP radiographs (Figure 37-3).

This evaluation algorithm allows us to provide the appropriate treatment recommendations based on stability. For stable, nondisplaced Lisfranc ligament sprains, we recommend conservative management. Patients are immobilized with a cast for 2 weeks then converted to a walker boot with partial weight-bearing restrictions for an additional 4 weeks. Progression to full weight bearing is then encouraged with an orthotic arch support.

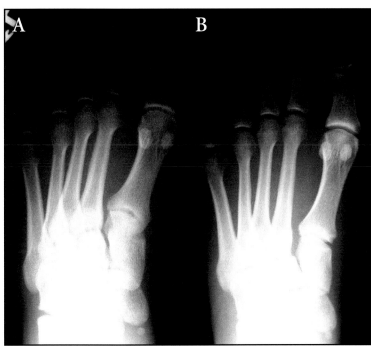

Figure 37-2. (A) Nonweight-bearing anteroposterior view of the uninjured side. (B) Weight-bearing AP view of the injured foot demonstrating diastasis of the 1-2 metatarsal space and malalignment of the second TMT joint.

In a 22-year-old football lineman with a displaced Lisfranc injury, our recommendation is surgery. We consider displacements of 2 mm or greater to be unstable injuries.[4] Our recommended surgical intervention includes open reduction and rigid internal fixation with 3.5 cortical screws (Figure 37-4). Some authors describe percutaneous reduction techniques. Anatomic reduction is imperative to achieving an excellent long-term result, so we routinely visualize the reduction through an open procedure. We prefer screw fixation over Kirschner wires, especially in heavy individuals, in order to maintain reduction and potentially facilitate a faster postoperative rehabilitation. Patients are placed in a nonweight-bearing cast for 6 weeks and then progressed to partial weight-bearing for 6 weeks in a walker boot. Full weight bearing is then initiated with a goal of routine screw removal at 4 months. Athletes may then gradually return to sport with an orthotic. Full return to sport may be delayed up to 1 year in more severe injuries.

Alternative management approaches for minimally displaced or ligamentous Lisfranc injuries range from conservative management to fusion. It is important to consider patient goals and expectations when suggesting a management protocol. If conservative management is chosen in a displaced injury, the ability to return to full sport participation may be less likely due to chronic instability and pain, and subsequent post-traumatic arthritis. On the other end of the spectrum, primary fusion in our opinion is overly aggressive in an acute injury in an athlete. The idea of primary fusion for a ligamentous Lisfranc injury has been popularized by Ly and Coetzee in a prospective randomized study.[5] A subsequent publication by the same authors warned against liberal use of fusion, commenting specifically on Lisfranc injuries seen in football players, where open reduction and internal fixation may be a better option.[6]

Another important variable to consider is the time from initial injury. It is not uncommon for these injuries to be misdiagnosed initially and present late to an orthopedic

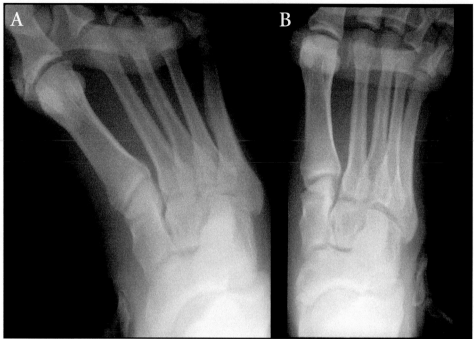

Figure 37-3. (A) Pre-stress view showing an intact medial column line. (B) Abduction stress view demonstrating disruption of the medial column line.

Figure 37-4. Open reduction and internal fixation of an unstable Lisfranc ligament complex injury.

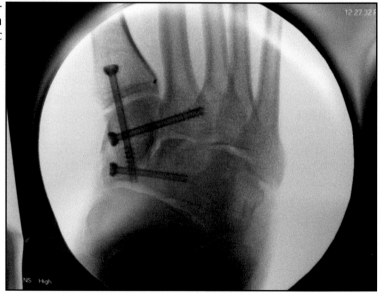

surgeon for treatment. The optimal management of unstable subacute or chronic Lisfranc ligament injuries in athletes is less clear. In general, we recommend open reduction and internal fixation whenever possible. Fusion may be a better option in neglected cases where significant arthritic changes are already present.

References

1. Nunley JA, Vertullo CJ. Classification, investigation, and management of midfoot sprains. *Am J Sports Med.* 2002;30:871-878.
2. Meyer SA, Callaghan JJ, Albright JP, et al. Midfoot sprains in collegiate football players. *Am J Sports Med.* 1994;22:392-401.
3. Raikin SM, Elias I, Dheer S, Besser MP, Morrison WB, Zoga AC. Prediction of midfoot instability in the subtle Lisfranc injury. Comparison of magnetic resonance imaging with intraoperative findings. *J Bone Joint Surg Am.* 2009;91:892-899.
4. Shapiro MS, Wascher DC, Finerman GA. Rupture of Lisfranc's ligament in athletes. *Am J Sports Med.* 1994;22:687-691.
5. Ly TV, Coetzee JC. Treatment of primary ligamentous Lisfranc joint injuries. Primary arthrodesis compared with open reduction and internal fixation. A prospective, randomized study. *J Bone Joint Surg Am.* 2006;88A:514-520.
6. Coetzee JC, Thuan VL. Treatment of primary ligamentous Lisfranc joint injuries: primary arthrodesis compared with open reduction and internal fixation. Surgical technique. *J Bone Joint Surg Am.* 2007;89A:122-127.

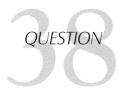

WHICH LATERAL TALAR PROCESS FRACTURES SHOULD I FIX?

Brian C. Toolan, MD

Historically, lateral process fractures of the talus were considered rare injuries and were fixed when they were displaced at least 2 mm. This amount of displacement implied that the fracture was unstable and unlikely to heal without an anatomical reduction and internal fixation. With the advent of snowboarding, the incidence of this injury has increased and more attention has been paid to understanding its natural history. Although little evidence exists to guide decision making, recent clinical and biomechanical investigations have provided useful information to bear in mind when deciding whether lateral process fractures should be treated with open reduction internal fixation.[1,2]

I consider several factors when I decide whether to fix, excise, or nonoperatively treat a lateral process of the talus fracture. Small (2 to 3 mm) nondisplaced fractures of the anterolateral corner of the lateral process represent bony avulsions of the lateral talofibular ligament. In my experience, these fractures do not benefit from surgery and reliably heal when the fracture is diagnosed and immobilized shortly after injury. Nondisplaced fractures of a larger size have been treated without surgery in the past; however, a recent cadaveric study demonstrated that a 1 cm^3 fragment involves all 3 of the major lateral stabilizing ligaments of the ankle (lateral talofibular, anterior talofibular, and posterior talofibular ligaments).[3] Thus, larger fragments should be closely evaluated for rotation and displacement. A computed tomography (CT) scan may assist in accurately determining the position of the fracture fragment. Also, a cast instead of a walker boot may provide increased immobilization to prevent late movement of a nondisplaced fragment.

I routinely fix most displaced fractures, but the size of the fragment(s) and the degree of comminution may necessitate excision of the fracture (Figure 38-1). I consider displacement and/or articular step-off or gapping of the fragment more than 1 to 2 mm unacceptable and indicative of an impending malunion or nonunion that will result in pain, stiffness, and loss of function. Furthermore, I believe the abnormal contact stresses during weight bearing that occur as a result of a malunion will lead to early degeneration

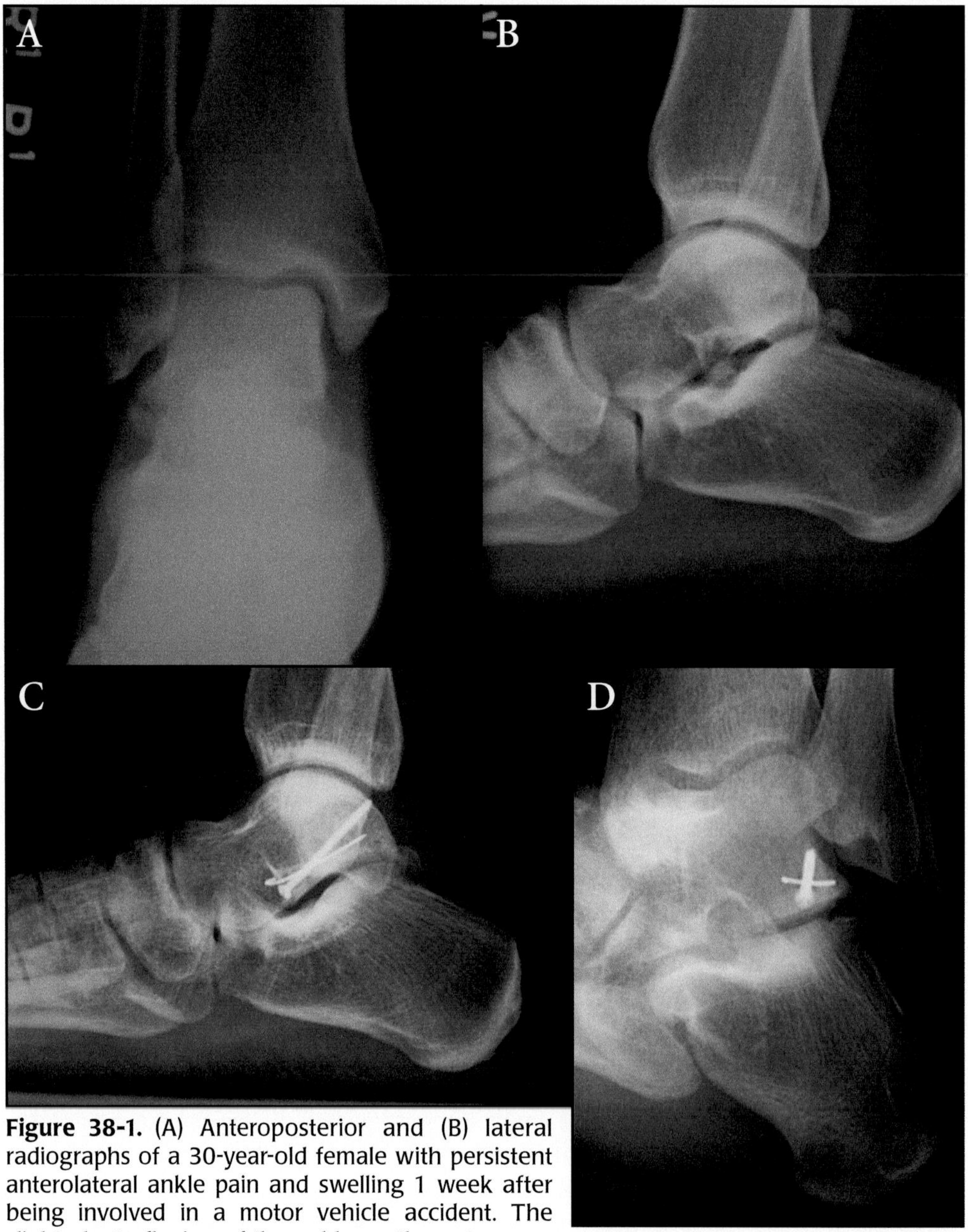

Figure 38-1. (A) Anteroposterior and (B) lateral radiographs of a 30-year-old female with persistent anterolateral ankle pain and swelling 1 week after being involved in a motor vehicle accident. The slight plantarflexion of the ankle on the anteroposterior view allows the lateral process fracture to be identified. The lateral view demonstrates the anteroinferior displacement of the fragment. (C) The lateral and (D) Broden's view radiographs obtained 3 months after open treatment demonstrating complete union of the anatomical reduction stabilized with a 2.7-mm cortical lag screw and a Kirschner wire. The Broden's view also demonstrates a healed impaction fracture of the anterolateral calcaneus.

of the subtalar joint. I will excise the fragment(s) if an anatomical reduction and stable fixation cannot be achieved because an iatrogenic malunion or nonunion will also lead to symptomatic early-onset arthrosis.

In my experience, fragments under 1 cm and very comminuted fractures are not amenable to satisfactory reduction and fixation. If the fragment cannot accept a fixation construct of at least a screw with a minimum diameter of 2.0 mm and a Kirschner wire, I do not believe that sufficient fixation has been achieved to permit early (1 to 2 weeks after surgery) range of motion. Without the initiation of early joint motion, the benefit of open treatment is obviated and the patient is better served with excision of the fragment. A biomechanical study has demonstrated that the excision of a 1-cm^3 fragment does not result in ankle or subtalar instability when assessed with stress radiographs.[3]

Comminuted fractures with impacted articular fragment(s) present the greatest challenge to successful reduction and fixation. The ability to restore, maintain, and assess articular congruity intraoperatively is the biggest obstacle in evaluating the acceptability of open treatment. In order to reduce an impacted, centrally located articular fragment(s), the cortical rim fragment(s) must be booked open while maintaining the ligamentous attachments. After the articular fragment is reduced, cancellous bone grafting often is necessary to maintain the reduction. Difficulties arise with visualizing the reduction of the cortical rim fragment(s) with these articular fragment(s). The anatomy of the sinus tarsi and the convex-concave articulation of subtalar joint may block the direct inspection of this step of the reduction. The placement of a small joint distractor and fluoroscopy with multiple Broden's views may assist with the intraoperative assessment of the articular surface. If the articular fragment(s) have a damaged or delaminated articular surface, I excise them and attempt to reduce the cortical rim fragment(s). If the articular cartilage of the calcaneus beneath the talar articular fragment is delaminated or absent, I excise the talar fragment. Under these 2 circumstances, it is unlikely that a smooth gliding articulation across the joint will be restored and pain with focal arthrosis will ensue rapidly. The clinical outcomes of this approach are not fully understood; however, a recent retrospective study found the presence of mild or moderate degenerative changes of the subtalar joint in 45% of patients with surgically treated fractures and an associated chondral injury.[1]

Overall, the effective evaluation and treatment of lateral process of the talus fractures begins with a high index of suspicion for traumatized patients presenting with anterolateral ankle pain. A detailed physical examination and thorough review of the radiographs and CT images will facilitate a complete characterization of the particular fracture. Careful consideration of the size, displacement, comminution, and location will lead to the most appropriate management of the fracture.

References

1. Valderrabano V, Perrn T, Ryf C, Rilmann P, Hinterman B. Snowboarder's talus fracture: treatment outcome of 20 cases after 3.5 years. *Am J Sports Med.* 2005;33:871-880.
2. vonKnoch F, Reckord U, vonKnoch M, Sommer C. Fracture of the lateral process of the talus in snowboarders. *J Bone Joint Surg.* 2007;89B:772-777.
3. Langer P, Nickisch F, Spenciner PE, Fleming B, DiGiovanni CW. In vitro evaluation of the effect of lateral process talar excision on ankle and subtalar joint stability. *Foot Ankle Int.* 2007;28:78-83.

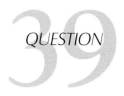

WHICH CALCANEUS FRACTURES SHOULD I OPERATE ON?

Pradeep Kodali, MD and Anand Vora, MD

Calcaneus fractures continue to be a difficult injury to manage. This chapter will focus on the treatment of intra-articular calcaneus fractures. There are extra-articular types, such as anterior process or tuberosity fractures, that we will briefly mention in the discussion of operative indications. In general, intra-articular calcaneus fractures involve a high-energy, axial load mechanism. The lateral process of the talus acts as a wedge driving into the calcaneus, which leads to a predictable fracture pattern. This often leads to intra-articular displacement of the posterior facet of the subtalar joint and calcaneocuboid joint and loss of the normal axial width and height of the calcaneus.

In order to determine which calcaneus fractures require surgery, an understanding of the basic radiographic relationships is critical. Two radiographic parameters that require evaluation are Bohler's angle and the crucial angle of Gissane. Both are evaluated on the lateral view. Bohler's angle is determined by drawing a line from the highest point on the anterior process of calcaneus to the highest point of the posterior facet and a second line drawn along the superior edge of the tuberosity (Figure 39-1). The normal value is 20 to 40 degrees, with a decrease indicating collapse of the posterior facet. The critical angle of Gissane is formed by a line along the lateral margin of the posterior facet and another line extending anterior to the beak of the calcaneus (Figure 39-2). The normal value is 95 to 105 degrees with an increase representing posterior facet collapse. Additional imaging views that are useful include a Harris axial view and Broden's views. A Harris axial view is useful in determining varus or valgus malalignment of the tuberosity, and Broden's views are useful in viewing the subtalar joint.

Computed tomography scan imaging is required to access the personality and extent of involvement of intra-articular calcaneus fractures. This should be performed using thin cuts with coronal and sagittal reconstructions. The Sanders classification (Table 39-1) is an extremely useful system for determining operative treatment and prognosis after fixation. The classification consists of separating the posterior facet into 3 separate fragments with the sustentaculum tali as the fourth constant fragment.

General operative indications for calcaneus fractures can be summarized in Table 39-2.

Figure 39-1. Lateral view depicting Bohler's angle.

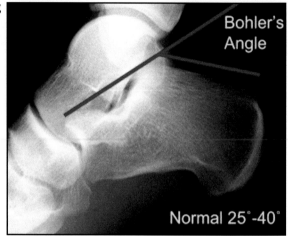

Figure 39-2. Lateral view depicting Gissane's angle.

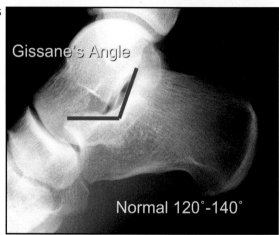

Table 39-1

Sanders Classification

Type 1	All nondisplaced articular fractures (less than 2 mm)
Type II	Two-part fractures of the posterior facet
Types IIA, IIB, IIIC	Based on location of primary fracture line
Type III	Three-part fractures usually featuring a centrally depressed fragment
Types IIIAB, IIIAC, IIIBC	Based on location of primary fracture line
Type IV	Four-part articular fractures

Table 39-2

Operative Indications for Calcaneus Fractures

- All open fractures
- Anterior process fractures with >25% involvement of calcaneocuboid joint
- Beak fractures that place the posterior skin at risk
- Displaced intra-articular fractures of posterior facet
- Fracture dislocations
- Irreducible body fractures with >30 degree varus or 40 degrees valgus deformity
- Lateral or medial process fractures with >1.5 cm displacement

Initial descriptions of surgical results were poor secondary to a high incidence of wound complications and malreduction, but newer open reduction, internal fixation (ORIF) techniques have lead to improved results. The key to improved outcomes with surgery relate to the ability to obtain an anatomic reduction of joint surfaces. The degree of initial fracture severity also correlates with results. A high learning curve should be recognized in the treatment of these injuries.

According to Buckley et al, patients with Bohler's angle <10 degrees, comminuted fracture patterns, large initial joint step-off, women, non-workman's compensation cases, and younger patients (age <29) have improved outcomes with surgery.[1] We have found these guidelines to be accurate in our practice; in addition, we prefer surgical reconstruction in patients with any amount of intra-articular step-off, significant axial malalignment causing peroneal tendon impairments, nerve impingement such as tarsal tunnel syndrome, sagittal height loss, greater than 5 degrees of tuberosity malalignment, and even in elderly patients. We believe that if wound complications can be avoided, restoration of the normal anatomical shape and alignment of the hindfoot and restoration of articular congruency results in optimal outcomes. We have found that the single most predictable factor in achieving a satisfactory outcome with surgical treatment is restoration of Bohler's angle, which generally implies that the above goals have been achieved (Figure 39-3).

For patients with Sanders Type IV fracture patterns, we prefer ORIF with primary subtalar arthrodesis in order to achieve the same goals as stated above (Figure 39-4). The benefit lies in restoring the anatomical alignment of the heel and allowing for a single recovery by fusing the subtalar joint during the index procedure.

Relative contraindications for surgery include nondisplaced fractures, fractures in diabetics with significant peripheral vascular disease, or elderly, household ambulators, and smokers. According to Buckley et al, patients older than 50, males, and those who are receiving workers' compensation and have an occupation involving a heavy workload should be treated without surgery.[1] In our practice, we consider the contraindications to be very flexible and soft. We place the greatest importance in the status of the soft tissues and ability to achieve tobacco cessation in smokers in an attempt to prevent complications. Age is really not a significant factor in determining operative versus nonoperative treatment in our practice.

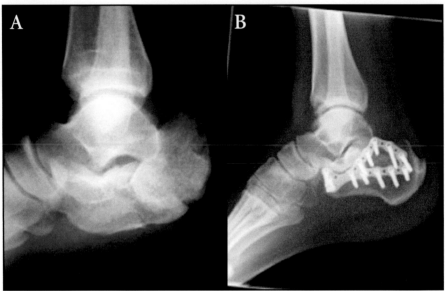

Figure 39-3. (A) Preoperative image showing calcaneus fracture with depressed posterior facet. (B) Postoperative view after ORIF and restoration of Bohler's angle.

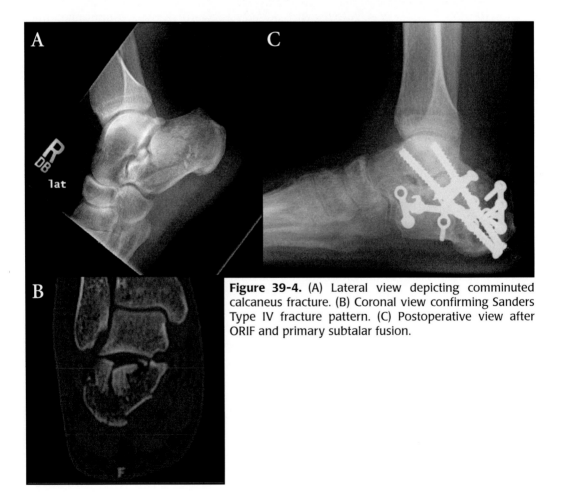

Figure 39-4. (A) Lateral view depicting comminuted calcaneus fracture. (B) Coronal view confirming Sanders Type IV fracture pattern. (C) Postoperative view after ORIF and primary subtalar fusion.

Nonoperative treatment primarily consists of a bulky dressing until soft tissue conditions have optimized, followed by boot immobilization, nonweight bearing for 10 to 12 weeks, and a physical therapy program focused on the preservation of subtalar motion and strengthening.

Operative treatment generally is performed via a standard extensile L-shaped lateral incision for exposure and reduction. For tongue-type fractures and for select intra-articular fractures, a percutaneous minimally invasive technique may be considered. External fixation techniques may be considered for an additional subset of patients who have strong radiographic surgical indications but soft tissue conditions when other relative contraindications are present, preventing the ability to perform open procedures. The description of such surgical techniques is beyond the scope of this chapter.

Reference

1. Buckley R, Tough S, McCormack R, et al. Operative compared with nonoperative treatment of displaced intra-articular calcaneal fractures: a prospective, randomized controlled multicenter trial. *J Bone Joint Surg Am.* 2002;84:1733-1744.

Suggested Readings

Sanders R. Intra-articular fractures of the calcaneus: present state of the art. *J Orthop Trauma.* 1992;6(2):252-265.

Sanders R, Clare M. Fractures of the calcaneus. In: Bucholz RW, Heckman JD, Court-Brown CM, Tornetta P, eds. *Rockwood and Green's Fractures in Adults.* Philadelphia, PA: Lippincott Williams & Wilkins; 2005:2293-2329.

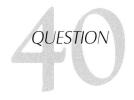

How Should I Fix My Patient With Multiple Metatarsal Fractures?

Simon Lee, MD and Samuel McArthur, MD

One of the things to remember is that not all metatarsal fractures are the same. It is important to understand the "personality" of the fracture and determine if there is intrinsic stability of the particular fracture pattern that you are evaluating.

The forefoot acts as a large base for load sharing with approximately two-thirds of body weight during the stance phase of gait, with the hallux generally carrying twice the load of each lesser metatarsal. They are well-fixed proximally both to the tarsals and each other by a series of dorsal, central, and plantar ligaments. Distally, the transverse intermetatarsal ligaments connect the plantar plates at the level of the metatarsal neck. Due to these constraints, isolated metatarsal fractures tend to be stable and rarely require operative intervention. Distal metatarsal neck fractures are an exception and may require fixation if significantly displaced due to absence of any soft tissue constraints.

When multiple metatarsals are fractured, constraint is lost and the distal fragments are typically pulled plantar and lateral by the toe flexors and interosseous muscles. Multiple metatarsal fractures occur both as a result of direct crushing injuries and indirect forces such as a motor vehicle collision or fall from a height.[1] A history of mechanism is important to obtain because a high-energy injury makes us more alert to the possibility of compartment syndrome and Lisfranc variants. Examination of the foot should emphasize neurovascular status, swelling and compartment tension, and condition of the soft tissues. Particularly with multiple metatarsal fractures, due to the high energy and more likely displacement, attention to any significant skin tenting or pressure necrosis is imperative. Anteroposterior, oblique, and lateral radiographs of the foot should be weight bearing or simulated weight bearing with the plate pressed against the plantar surface of the foot whenever possible. Fractures of the base of the metatarsal, particularly of the second, frequently represent a Lisfranc injury and a high index of suspicion is required. Additionally, the third metatarsal is rarely fractured in isolation and multiple metatarsal fractures are always contiguous. We closely scrutinize adjacent metatarsals if we believe we have encountered an injury that violates these tenets. As a result of the rare occurrence of isolated second and third metatarsal fractures, a subsequent ligamentous injury to the adjacent tarsometatarsal joint is present until proven otherwise. A magnetic resonance imaging scan is helpful when the diagnosis or extent of the soft tissue injury is unclear, especially in the presented case. In cases where multiple fractures are present, we would otherwise prefer a computed tomography scan.

There are no critically evaluated criteria for determining what represents unacceptable displacement of metatarsal fractures, although the guidelines set forth by Armagan and Sherref of less than 10 degrees of sagittal angulation or 3 to 4 mm of displacement in any plane are frequently referenced.[2] In general, the fourth and fifth tarsometatarsal joints are more mobile and these metatarsals can probably tolerate greater degrees of sagittal deformity. As well, some authors cite concern of interdigital neuroma with closing of the intermetatarsal distance; however, we have rarely noted this to be an issue. We have found it more helpful to consider restoration of equal distribution of weight among the lesser metatarsal heads to prevent future transfer metatarsalgia lesions as the primary goal of treatment.[3] This requires minimal displacement in the sagittal plane to prevent increased pressure from plantarflexion or transfer pressure to adjacent metatarsals from dorsiflexion as well as approximation of the normal cascade. Occasionally, we will encounter metatarsal base fractures or nondisplaced fractures that meet these criteria more distally and will treat them in a hard-soled shoe or short Controlled Ankle Movement (CAM) boot with weight bearing as tolerated through the heel for 4 to 6 weeks with radiographs taken on a biweekly basis. Fractures occurring more distally in the shaft or neck of the metatarsal tend to progressively displace. We have not found closed reduction without fixation to be successful in maintaining alignment. We treat displaced distal fractures, fractures with unacceptable initial displacement, and fractures that are open or are associated with compartment syndrome operatively.

Most fractures can be treated with closed reduction and percutaneous pinning with a 2.0-mm Kirschner wire (K-wire). The usual plantar and lateral displacement is reversed with manual traction on the digits followed by pressure on the plantar and dorsal surface of the metatarsal. Occasionally, a small pointed reduction clamp or elevator inserted percutaneously can be helpful for correcting residual displacement. The toe is dorsiflexed at the metatarsophalangeal (MTP), and we insert a K-wire retrograde from the plantar surface of the foot through the metatarsal head and shaft, gaining purchase proximally in the metatarsal base. Alternatively, the K-wire can be started antegrade at the fracture site and driven out of the plantar distal aspect of the foot while the MTP is dorsiflexed. The fracture is then reduced and the K-wire driven back retrograde into the metatarsal base. For segmental fractures or cases in which we cannot achieve an acceptable closed reduction, we will use a longitudinal web space incision to expose the fracture sites. At this point, we will make a decision to drive K-wires under direct reduction and visualization versus internal fixation with mini fragment fixation. For severely comminuted fractures, supplemental transverse intermetatarsal K-wires can be used to assist in maintaining length. Incisions should be strategically placed, particularly in the setting of compartment syndrome or open injury to allow the greatest number of procedures with the least amount of soft tissue trauma and retraction possible. We have not found it necessary to routinely include the base of the proximal phalanx with longitudinal pinning or to use multiple wires to control rotation, as advocated by some authors.

Alternate methods of fixation include mini fragment screws with or without plates. Infrequently, we have used 2 mini fragment (2.0 or 2.7 mm) screws to fix long

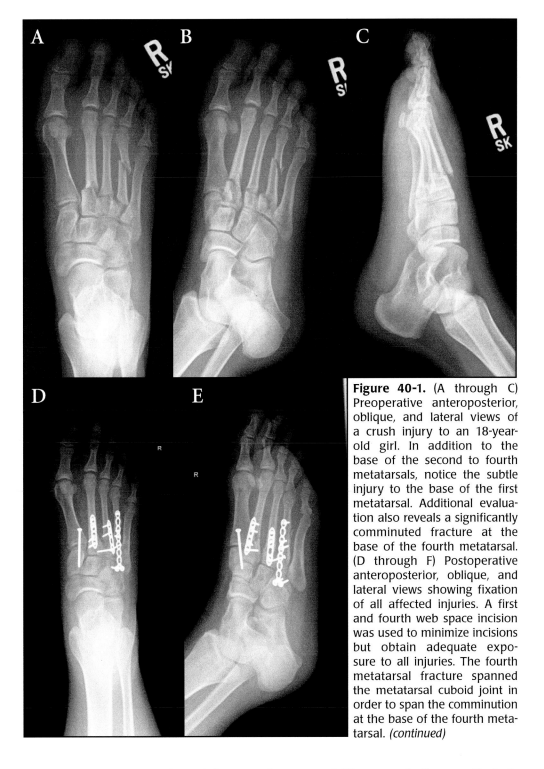

Figure 40-1. (A through C) Preoperative anteroposterior, oblique, and lateral views of a crush injury to an 18-year-old girl. In addition to the base of the second to fourth metatarsals, notice the subtle injury to the base of the first metatarsal. Additional evaluation also reveals a significantly comminuted fracture at the base of the fourth metatarsal. (D through F) Postoperative anteroposterior, oblique, and lateral views showing fixation of all affected injuries. A first and fourth web space incision was used to minimize incisions but obtain adequate exposure to all injuries. The fourth metatarsal fracture spanned the metatarsal cuboid joint in order to span the comminution at the base of the fourth metatarsal. *(continued)*

oblique fractures, most often of the second metatarsal. However, similar to a fibula fracture, we believe a neutralizing plate allows for earlier weight bearing and mobilization (Figure 40-1). We have also used mini fragment plate and screw constructs to bridge

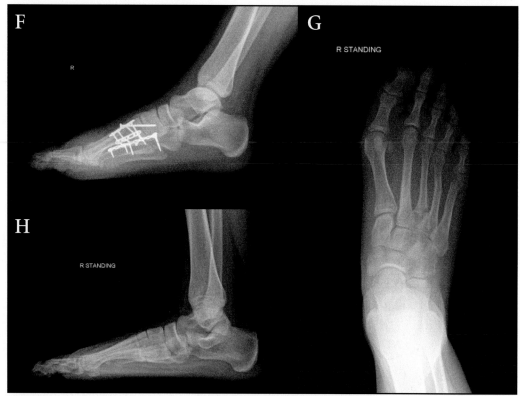

Figure 40-1 (continued). (G, H) AP and lateral radiographs with hardware removed. Note the restoration of the bony anatomy and the metatarsal head cascade.

comminution in fractures with sufficient bone stock proximally and distally. We have recently found that in fractures in which the soft tissue envelope is at risk, the use of mini external fixators specifically for the border metatarsals (first and fifth) has been extremely useful for either temporizing the fracture or even definitive fixation (Figure 40-2). Oftentimes, these fixators can also be used to span comminuted fractures at the base of these fractures to the adjacent cuneiform or cuboid.

Postoperatively, if there is external hardware, we maintain a nonweight-bearing status until we remove the pins and/or the fixator in the office at 4 to 6 weeks. If we perform an open reduction, internal fixation, we maintain the same protocol as for nonoperative treatment: a short CAM boot with weight bearing as tolerated through the heel for 4 to 6 weeks with radiographs taken on a biweekly basis. Bioabsorbable pins obviate the need for implant removal; however, we have found they are not rigid enough in these settings to provide adequate stability.

In general, we have found it to be true that good results can be expected with careful soft tissue handling and restoration of sagittal balance, although the prognosis for severely comminuted or open injuries remains more guarded. Essentially, we feel that the treatment of the weight-bearing foot should encompass all of the tools that orthopedists are familiar with and trained to use to obtain an acceptable reduction in order to allow earlier mobilization and prevent future complications.

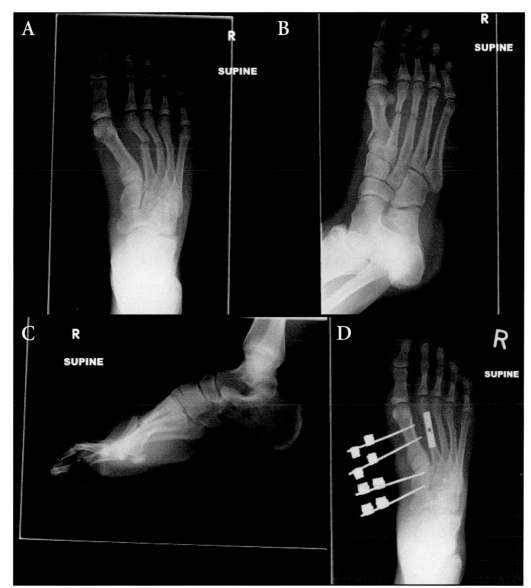

Figure 40-2. (A through C) Preoperative anteroposterior, lateral, and oblique views showing an unstable and displaced fracture pattern with significant first metatarsal comminution and angulation, and the significant dorsal angulation on the lateral view of the second metatarsal. (D through F) Postoperative radiographs showing correction of angulation and shortening of the first metatarsal with the use of a mini-external fixator device. Fixation of the second metatarsal was performed with a small fragment one-third tubular plate. Note the indirect correction of the third and fourth metatarsal fractures due to the pull of the transverse intermetatarsal ligaments. *(continued)*

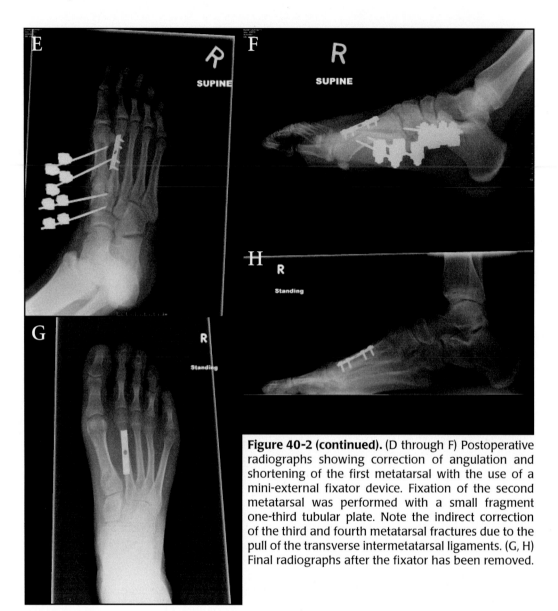

Figure 40-2 (continued). (D through F) Postoperative radiographs showing correction of angulation and shortening of the first metatarsal with the use of a mini-external fixator device. Fixation of the second metatarsal was performed with a small fragment one-third tubular plate. Note the indirect correction of the third and fourth metatarsal fractures due to the pull of the transverse intermetatarsal ligaments. (G, H) Final radiographs after the fixator has been removed.

References

1. Petrisor BA, Ekrol I, Court-Brown C. The epidemiology of metatarsal fractures. *Foot Ankle Int.* 2006;27(3):172-174.
2. Armagan OE, Sherref MJ. Injuries to the toes and metatarsals. *Orthop Clin North Am.* 2001;32(1):1-10.
3. Sánchez Alepuz E, Vicent Carsi V, Alcántara P, Llabrés AJ. Fractures of the central metatarsal. *Foot Ankle Int.* 1996:17(4):200-203.

WHAT IS YOUR DECISION-MAKING PROCESS FOR PILON FRACTURES?

Sameer J. Lodha, MD and Walter W. Virkus, MD

The initial evaluation and subsequent management of pilon fractures is driven by 2 overriding goals—the anatomic repair of the articular surface, and the preservation of a viable soft tissue envelope.[1] To this end, we recommend the following approach to these often severe injuries.

First, the mechanism of injury should be identified. Low-energy injuries are usually torsional, with larger fracture fragments. High-energy injuries are usually from axial loading and have a wide range of severity.[1] A high-energy pilon fracture requires an assessment of the proximal limbs and the axial skeleton to identify any other associated injuries.

Next, the soft tissue envelope is evaluated. The quality of the soft tissues is of paramount importance in the treatment of pilon fractures and will dictate the timing of any operative repair.[2] Open fractures require expeditious irrigation and débridement. Closed fractures with significant deformity can lead to ongoing soft tissue injury and are an indication for urgent closed reduction. As part of this evaluation, compartments are assessed with regular monitoring for signs of impending compartment syndrome.[3]

Imaging studies are then obtained. Plain radiographs including anteroposterior, lateral, and mortise views will allow a careful assessment of the injury (Figure 41-1). These complex injuries often require computed tomography (CT) scans for further elucidation of fracture anatomy; however, we prefer to wait until after the application of a spanning external fixator prior to obtaining advanced imaging because the spatial relationship of fracture fragments may change significantly with partial reduction achieved with ligamentotaxis.

Imaging studies will allow classification of the injury and help complete identification of indications for operative treatment. The Arbeitsgemeinschaft für Osteosynthesefragen/Orthopaedic Trauma Association classification is inclusive and detailed and is thus useful for both descriptive and planning purposes. This classification system divides distal tibial injuries into 3 major groups: type A is extra-articular; type B is partial articular; and type C is complete involvement of the articular surface. Displacement of greater than

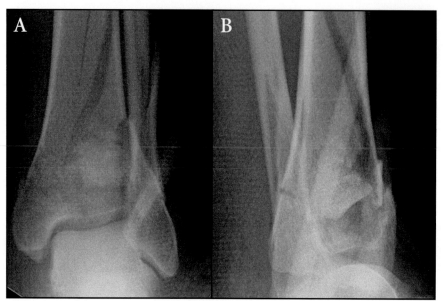

Figure 41-1. (A) Anteroposterior and (B) lateral radiographs of a pilon fracture, demonstrating intra-articular depression.

2 to 3 mm of any articular fragment is an indication for operative repair in most circumstances. Other indications are evidence of joint instability, open fracture, malalignment, and vascular injury. Nonoperative management is essentially limited to patients with nondisplaced fractures or a poor medical prognosis.

The initial operative management of these fractures should include the application of a spanning external fixator, possibly with internal fixation of the fibula, preferably within 12 to 18 hours of the injury. In the setting of an open fracture, this is combined with a thorough irrigation and débridement. Once an external fixator is in place, it is reasonable to delay further surgical treatment for 7 to 20 days in order to allow recovery of the soft tissues.

External fixation confers substantial benefits. It allows an initial reduction of fracture fragments via ligamentotaxis, thereby aiding in soft tissue recovery and preventing soft tissue contracture (Figure 41-2). Additionally, this provisional alignment makes definitive reduction and fixation much easier. It also permits early mobilization of the patient, reducing the risks associated with prolonged bed rest. Internal fixation of the fibula assists in maintaining length across the fracture (again helping prevent soft tissue contracture), restores the rotational alignment of the fibula, and improves reduction of tibial fragments through ligamentotaxis. Possible disadvantages of fibular plating include compromising future incisions and malreducing the fibula, which can hinder reduction of the tibia. These risks can be minimized through judicious surgical planning and meticulous reduction. In the setting of open fractures, efforts can be made to use existing wounds to access the fibula. The posterolateral approach to the fibula is often used as it permits easy access to the fibula while also helping maintain an adequate skin bridge in the event an anteromedial or even anterolateral approach is used for later tibial fixation. In the setting of an open fracture, these immediate interventions can be augmented with placement of

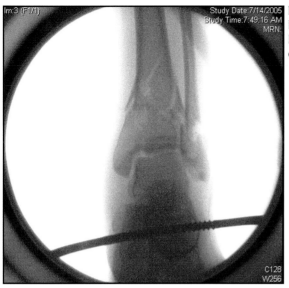

Figure 41-2. Intraoperative fluoroscopic image of fracture seen in Figure 41-5. Intraoperative distraction permits significant fracture reduction via ligamentotaxis.

antibiotic beads. Closure of any incision should be with a tension-free suture; alternatively, a wound vac or bead pouch can be used. Patients can then be discharged home with strict instructions to keep the injured extremity elevated and adequate pain control in place.

Once this first stage fixation has been completed, a CT scan can be obtained to elucidate fracture anatomy, especially in regard to the articular surface. Typically, CT scans of pilon fractures will help identify the following major fragments: the Tillaux-Chaput (anterolateral) fragment, the Volkmann's (posterior) fragment, the medial malleolus, and the remaining articular surface (die-punch), which may show a range in severity of comminution. Given that there can be significant variability in the articular fragment pattern, the information from CT scans is key in adequate preoperative planning.[4]

The patient should thereafter be re-examined at 5- to 7-day intervals to assess the wound for signs of infection, cessation of any drainage, and resolution of edema and fracture blisters. Once the soft tissue envelope is deemed ready, we proceed with definitive fixation. The main considerations at this point are regarding the surgical approach and the type of fixation to be used.

The main approaches for treatment of pilon fractures are anteromedial and anterolateral. Posterolateral and posteromedial approaches can be used, usually as supplemental approaches. The optimal approach is driven by the need to obtain an anatomic reduction of articular fragments. This reduction is aided by distraction and ligamentotaxis obtained by using the previously applied external fixator pins. Reduction of the central comminution and posterior fragment is usually accomplished by working through the "window" afforded by the anterior fracture and Chaput fragment (Figure 41-3). Typically, we will use an anterolateral approach if the Chaput fragment is small (less than half the width of the anterior cortex; Figure 41-4) and an anteromedial approach if the Chaput fragment is large (Figure 41-5). The ultimate choice of surgical approach is also influenced by the need to maintain an adequate skin bridge from any open wound or previous incision used for fibular plating.[5,6]

Figure 41-3. Anterolateral approach to the fracture seen in Figures 41-1 and 41-4, demonstrating excellent view of primary fracture fragments.

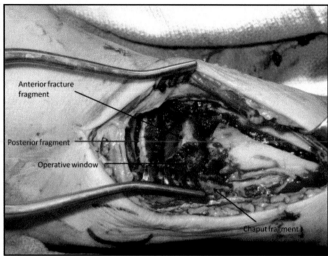

Figure 41-4. Axial CT image of the same fracture seen in Figure 41-1. A small anterolateral fragment is seen, lending this fracture to an anterolateral approach.

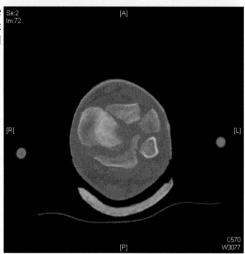

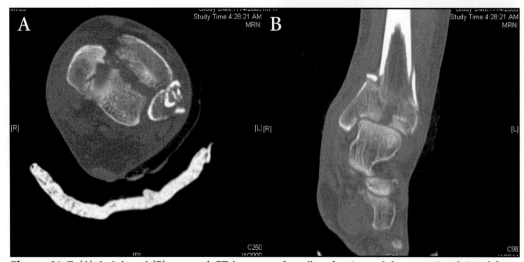

Figure 41-5. (A) Axial and (B) coronal CT images of a pilon fracture. A large anterolateral fragment is present. In this case, the anteromedial approach will be optimal for fragment visualization and reduction.

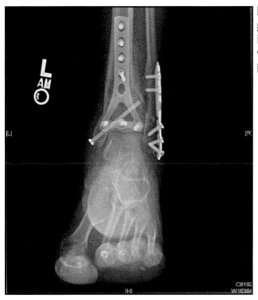

Figure 41-6. Six-month postoperative radiograph of patient in Figures 41-2 and 41-5, showing reduction of the articular surface and fixation via an anteromedial approach. Fracture healing is evident.

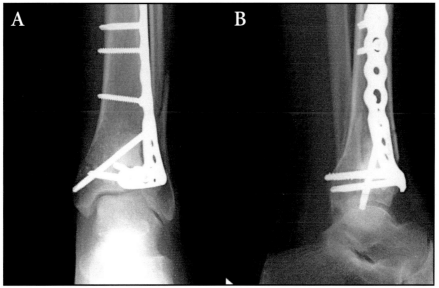

Figure 41-7. (A) Anteroposterior and (B) lateral images of fracture seen in Figures 41-1 and 41-4 after open reduction, internal fixation with an anterolateral precontoured locking plate.

Pilon fracture fixation consists of lag screws and plates. Large fragment plates are no longer routinely used due to hardware prominence; instead, one-third tubular plates, mini fragment plates, and other small fragment plates are used (Figure 41-6). It is sometimes necessary to use more than one plate; precontoured plates are available that work well for fixing the articular segment to the shaft (Figure 41-7).

In certain situations, an external fixator may be chosen as the definitive treatment. This may occur when the degree of comminution is such that plate fixation will not achieve a reduction superior to that achievable by ligamentotaxis. Other considerations that support the use of external fixation include a very poor soft tissue envelope and medical comorbidities, including smoking, diabetes, inflammatory arthritis, and chronic steroid use. All of these conditions would greatly increase the potential complications resulting from the soft tissue dissection required for open reduction, internal fixation.[7] When using an external fixator, attempts should still be made to reduce the articular fragments and stabilize them with lag screws.

Postoperatively, we keep patients touch-down weight bearing for 3 months. They may start active range of motion exercises 7 to 10 days from surgery. Final progression to weight bearing as tolerated can be made at 10 to 14 weeks provided there is further evidence of healing.

References

1. Borrelli J, Ellis E. Pilon fractures: assessment and treatment. *Orthop Clin North Am.* 2002;33(1):231-245.
2. Sirkin M, Sanders R, DiPasquale T, Herscovici D Jr. A staged protocol for soft tissue management in the treatment of complex pilon fractures. *J Orthop Trauma.* 2004;18(8 Suppl):S32-S38.
3. Gardner MJ, Mehta S, Barei DP, Nork SE. Treatment protocol for open AO/OTA type C3 pilon fractures with segmental bone loss. *J Orthop Trauma.* 2008;22(7):451-457.
4. Topliss CJ, Jackson M, Atkins RM. Anatomy of pilon fractures of the distal tibia. *J Bone Joint Surg Br.* 2005;87(5):692-697.
5. Borrelli J, Catalano L. Open reduction and internal fixation of pilon fractures. *J Orthop Trauma.* 1999;13:573-582.
6. Chen L, O'Shea K, Early JS. The use of medial and lateral surgical approaches for the treatment of tibial plafond fractures. *J Orthop Trauma.* 2007;21(3):207-211.
7. Marsh JL, Borrelli J Jr, Dirschl DR, Sirkin MS. Fractures of the tibial plafond. *Instr Course Lect.* 2007;56:331-352.

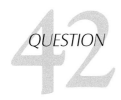

Do I Rod or Plate My Distal Third Tibia Fractures? Should I Fix the Fibula, Too?

Cara A. Cipriano, MD and Walter W. Virkus, MD

Fractures of the metaphyseal distal tibia are common but often difficult to manage. Reduction is not only more challenging to achieve and maintain than in midshaft fractures, but also more important in terms of clinical outcome. Whereas 5 degrees of varus/valgus angulation is considered tolerable in the shaft, the same deformity in the distal tibia can result in ankle pain and stiffness. Treatment of these injuries should be determined based on evaluation of the fracture pattern, the condition of the surrounding soft tissues, and the functional and rehabilitation goals of the individual patient.

Fractures that are minimally displaced or reducible with closed manipulation may be managed nonoperatively with either casting or functional bracing. Oblique or spiral fractures are inherently less stable and therefore more likely to angulate and shorten, which can lead to malunion. In addition, tibial fractures in which the fibula remains intact are predisposed to fall into varus angulation. Fractures that are treated nonoperatively must be followed closely with serial radiographs in order to ensure maintenance of the reduction. Adequate 3-point molding may be more difficult to achieve in obese patients, which may also lead to a higher incidence of displacement. Finally, casting may be contraindicated if significant damage to the surrounding soft tissues is present.

Cases in which the fracture itself or the surrounding tissues require stable fixation can be treated operatively using external fixation, intramedullary nailing, or plating. External fixators are typically reserved for high-energy injuries with significant soft tissue damage. Ankle spanning and nonspanning as well as thin-wire ring fixators are all reasonable options.

Plate fixation results in a lower incidence of malalignment, avoids the risk of anterior knee pain associated with intramedullary nailing,[1] and preserves the intramedullary blood supply. However, conventional open dissection violates the periosteum and surrounding tissues, potentially increasing the risk of nonunion and infection. This is somewhat less of a concern when minimally invasive plating techniques are employed, although anatomic reduction becomes more difficult because the fracture is not directly visualized.[2] Postoperatively, patients may complain of painful or prominent hardware,

Figure 42-1. Excellent alignment of a distal tibia fracture using open reduction, internal fixation (ORIF) from an anterolateral approach, which provides maximum soft tissue coverage of the plate.

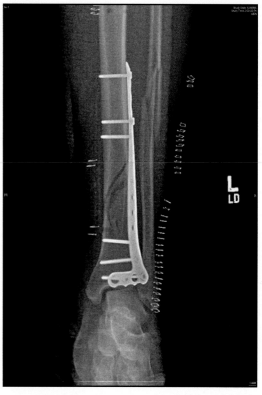

particularly if placed medially, but plate removal typically results in effective relief. Finally, anterolateral plating creates a better soft tissue envelope but does carry a risk of superficial peroneal nerve injury (Figure 42-1).

In cases of plate fixation, soft tissue-friendly surgical techniques should be employed to prevent wound complications and enhance fracture healing. Percutaneous forceps or distractors can be used to assist in reduction. Lag screws placed perpendicular to oblique fractures can be used to achieve compression, but only if anatomic reduction can be obtained. In most minimally invasive situations, reduction focuses on restoring length, alignment, and rotation, with a bridge plate construct that provides relative stability. Lag screws across the fracture should not be used in these cases as they impart absolute stability to a nonanatomic reduction, which can lead to nonunion. Percutaneous anterolateral fixation carries a high risk of both superficial and deep peroneal nerve injury and should be avoided. Anteromedial plating is easily done in a minimally invasive fashion, although this can lead to complications associated with hardware prominence. Percutaneous screws are placed, leaving an uninstrumented portion in the midpoint of the plate to allow a small amount of relative motion. The benefit of using locking screws has not been demonstrated, although they may improve stability in fractures with limited area for distal fixation.[3] If satisfactory reduction cannot be achieved using the minimally invasive technique, conventional open reduction and plating should be performed.

We usually prefer intramedullary nailing to plate fixation for the treatment of distal tibial shaft fractures. Intramedullary nailing establishes relative stability across the fracture site, thereby obviating the need for anatomic reduction and making this technique preferable in cases of comminuted fractures. In addition, decreased trauma to soft tissues

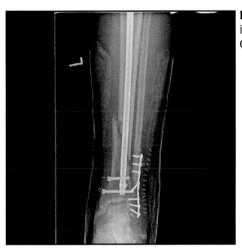

Figure 42-2. Residual valgus alignment despite intramedullary nail placement in the tibial shaft and ORIF of the fibula.

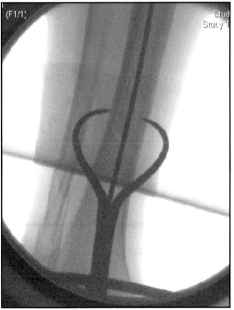

Figure 42-3. Intraoperative fluoroscopy image demonstrating anatomic reduction prior to nailing, achieved with a percutaneously placed clamp.

reduces the risk of wound complications and infection, and the load-sharing nail allows for earlier weight bearing than the load-bearing plate. The development of nails with multiplanar distal interlocking screws has lead to improved maintenance of rotational alignment and length, even in the absence of a tight endosteal fit. Finally, although nailing affects the intramedullary blood supply, this has not been shown to impair fracture healing.

Intramedullary nailing is more technically challenging in fractures of the distal tibia than the shaft. Because of the widening of the canal at the metaphysis, insertion of the nail does not ensure reduction of the fracture, and eccentric reaming can result from inadequate control of the distal fragment (Figure 42-2). In most circumstances, pointed clamps placed percutaneously can hold a reduction during the nailing process (Figure 42-3). I find the intraoperative placement of 2-pin external fixation, or travelling traction, particularly helpful in the difficult cases when the clamp is ineffective. To use

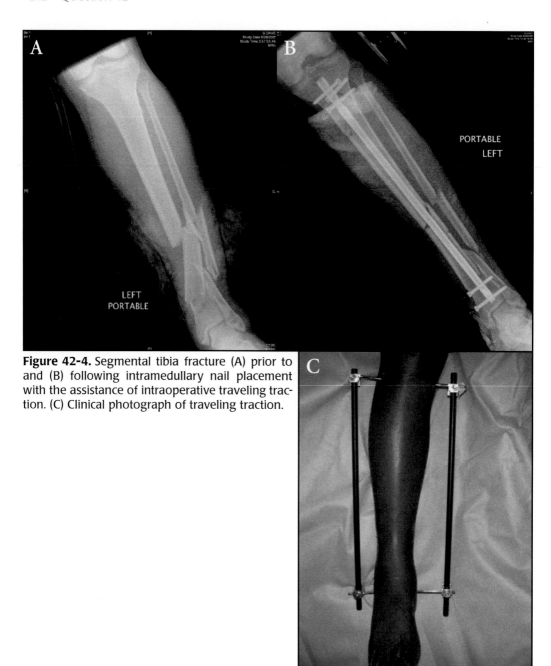

Figure 42-4. Segmental tibia fracture (A) prior to and (B) following intramedullary nail placement with the assistance of intraoperative traveling traction. (C) Clinical photograph of traveling traction.

this technique, a 5.0-mm centrally threaded transfixion pin is placed from lateral to medial through the metaphysis of the proximal tibia, making sure that it is posterior to the path of the nail. Careful dissection down to bone must be performed in order to avoid damaging the peroneal nerve as it courses anterior to the lateral malleolus. A second pin is placed medial to lateral in the distal tibial physeal scar, or, if the fracture is too distal, in the calcaneus. The 2 pins are then connected with the fixator bars in a rectangular configuration and adjusted to reduce the fracture (Figure 42-4). Manual manipulation

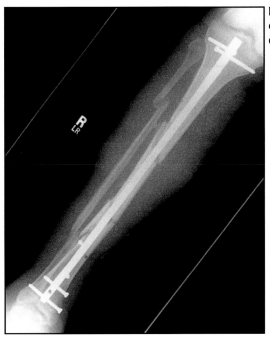

Figure 42-5. Final alignment achieved in a comminuted distal tibia fracture with the use of blocking screws.

and the use of a bump may also help. This technique has been shown to produce a low rate of postoperative malalignment.[4] Alternatives to traveling traction include the use of blocking screws, which can be placed adjacent to the desired path of the nail to direct its course. This effectively narrows the medullary canal, preventing deviation of the nail in the wide metaphyseal bone. Blocking screws are typically placed on the side of the tibia opposite the apex of the deformity (on the concave side of deformity) in order to counteract this deformity (Figure 42-5).

The treatment of associated distal fibula fractures remains controversial. Fibular plating has been associated with an increased rate of tibial malunion in patients who underwent intramedullary nailing.[1] In certain instances, however, fibular fixation may be helpful in realigning the tibia or improving the lateral stability of the leg.[5] Compelling indications for fibula fixation include open fractures and lateral malleolar fractures involving the articular surface of the ankle. Likewise, any associated medial or posterior malleolar fractures should be reduced and stabilized with screws in order to minimize the risk of post-traumatic ankle arthritis.

The most common complication of intramedullary nailing is anterior knee pain, which has been reported in greater than 50% of patients postoperatively. Careful attention to protecting the patellar tendon and the anterior intermeniscal ligament, as well as selection of the appropriate nail length, may reduce the incidence of this problem. The nail may be removed after stable healing has taken place, which improves symptoms in approximately half of patients.

Distal tibia fractures are a challenging injury. The surgeon should understand the risks, benefits, and difficulties of the treatment options. Many treatment options are associated with good patient outcomes if performed well.

References

1. Vallier HA, Le TT, Bedi A. Radiographic and clinical comparisons of distal tibia shaft fractures (4-11 cm proximal to the plafond): plating versus intramedullary nailing. *J Orthop Trauma.* 2008;22(5):307-311.
2. Collinge CA, Sanders RW. Percutaneous plating in the lower extremity. *J Am Acad Orthop Surg.* 2000;8:211-216.
3. Bedi A, Le TT, Karunakar MA. Surgical treatment of nonarticular distal tibia fractures. *J Am Acad Orthop Surg.* 2006;14:406-414.
4. Wysocki RW, Kapotas JS, Virkus WW. Intramedullary nailing of proximal and distal one-third tibial shaft fractures with intraoperative two-pin external fixation. *J Trauma.* 2009;66(4):1135-1139.
5. Egol KA, Weisz R, Hiebert R, et al. Does fibular plating improve alignment after intramedullary nailing or distal metaphyseal tibia fractures? *J Orthop Trauma.* 2006;20:94-103.

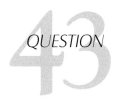
HOW DO YOU FIX YOUR SYNDESMOTIC INJURIES?
CAN I USE A TIGHTROPE NOW?

Jaymes D. Granata, MD and Terrence M. Philbin, DO

The diagnosis and management of ankle syndesmotic injuries have been the topic of much debate in recent years. As a key secondary stabilizer of the ankle joint (second to the deltoid ligament), the syndesmosis plays an integral role in ankle mechanics. Composed of the anterior inferior tibiofibular ligament, posterior inferior tibiofibular ligament, transverse ligament, and interosseous membrane, the syndesmosis secures the distal fibula into the incisura and provides lateral stability to the ankle mortise. Unstable injuries lead to diastasis between the distal tibia and fibula with a subsequent alteration of normal ankle motion.

Syndesmotic injuries occur both in isolation (high ankle sprain) or along with ankle fractures. Traditional teaching has associated these injuries with Weber C ankle fractures, but one should consider the possibility of a syndesmotic disruption in other fracture patterns as well. A recent clinical study reported a 39% incidence of syndesmotic instability in Weber B ankle fractures.[1]

There are a variety of fixation techniques described for stabilization of the syndesmosis, including screws (traditional and bioabsorbable), staples, thin wire fixators, Kirschner wires, syndesmotic hooks, and cerclage wires. Screw fixation is the most popular technique. The advantages of screw fixation include familiarity of use, low cost, and widespread availability. However, the syndesmosis is dynamic and allows for a certain degree of motion, so one disadvantage of screws is the rigid fixation that they provide. This overconstraint may lead to screw loosening, pullout, and breakage. Some surgeons also advocate routine screw removal, adding the potential morbidity of an additional surgical procedure.

The imperfections of screw fixation have led to the development of alternative dynamic fixation techniques, including the TightRope (Arthrex, Inc, Naples, FL). The TightRope is composed of a #5 FiberWire loop and 2 buttons. The device is tensioned to hold the syndesmotic reduction while allowing more physiologic movement at the distal tibiofibular joint. Proposed advantages of this technique include the elimination of a secondary procedure to remove the implant and earlier mobilization without the concern of screw failure.

Figure 43-1. Injury films demonstrating a Weber C ankle fracture with disruption of the syndesmosis.

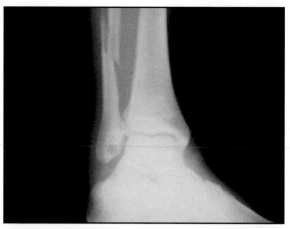

Figure 43-2. Highly unstable injury pattern with a widened medial joint space.

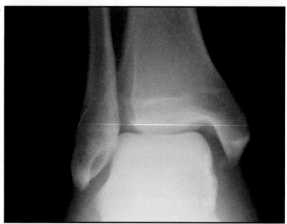

We generally use either screw or TightRope fixation to treat ankle syndesmotic injuries. Our decision is based on a number of factors, including patient age, weight, activity level, and time from injury. We have found the TightRope to be useful in both isolated soft tissue injuries as well as ankle fractures with syndesmotic diastasis. There have been reports of TightRope failure in highly unstable fracture patterns, including Maisonneuve type fractures. If a TightRope is to be used in these situations, we recommend using 2 TightRopes 1 cm apart in a divergent pattern to increase the stability of the construct (Figures 43-1 through 43-3). For diabetics, obese patients, and those with poor bone quality, we typically resort to rigid internal fixation with screws.

Our TightRope postoperative protocol includes 6 weeks of nonweight bearing in a splint/cast, followed by weight bearing as tolerated in a fracture boot. Ankle range of motion exercises are encouraged by week 3. Once full weight bearing is achieved in the fracture boot, patients are progressed to an athletic shoe with an ankle brace. When we use screw fixation, we follow a similar protocol, but the initial nonweight bearing is continued for a total of 10 weeks.

Favorable clinical outcomes have been reported using the TightRope for syndesmotic fixation.[2,3] As with any surgical implant or procedure, there are potential complications of which the surgeon and patient should be aware. We have seen 2 complications specific

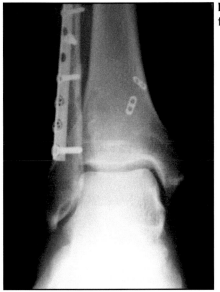

Figure 43-3. Open reduction and internal fixation of the fibula with syndesmotic fixation using 2 TightRopes.

to TightRope fixation, including a fracture of the lateral cortex of the fibula in one patient and skin irritation with local inflammatory reactions in multiple patients.

After the TightRope is tensioned, there is a stress riser at the button-bone interface due to the small surface area of the button. To better distribute the tensioning stress, we now routinely place the TightRope through a plate in both isolated ligament injuries and ankle fractures.

The local inflammatory response and skin irritation is likely due to a combination of factors, including knot prominence and the composition of the suture material itself. The FiberWire suture is coated with silicone and has been associated with a foreign body reaction in some cases, especially when placed in areas of high friction.[4] We recommend leaving a small tail after cutting the FiberWire suture and laying it flat to reduce the prominence of the knot.

Regardless of the type of fixation used, anatomic reduction and stable fixation is the key to achieving the best long-term outcome. It is important to be meticulous with your reduction. Malreduction rates have been reported as high as 52% using postoperative computed tomography scans.[5] Patients who have malreduced syndesmotic joints generally have a worse outcome due to persistent pain, instability, and ankle arthrosis.

The TightRope technique is a viable option with its own set of potential risks and benefits. No one fixation method has been found to be far superior to all the rest, and the ultimate decision for fixation of syndesmotic injuries depends on surgeon preference and familiarity.

References

1. Stark E, Tornetta P, Creevey WR. Syndesmotic instability in Weber B ankle fractures: a clinical evaluation. *J Orthop Trauma.* 2007;21(9):643-646.
2. Cottom JM, Hyer CF, Philbin TM, Berlet GC. Treatment of syndesmotic disruptions with the Arthrex TightRope: a report of 25 cases. *Foot Ankle Int.* 2008;29:773-780.

3. Thornes B, Shannon F, Guiney AM, Hession P, Masterson E. Suture-button syndesmosis fixation: accelerated rehabilitation and improved outcomes. *Clin Orthop Rel Res*. 2005;431:207-212.
4. Mack AW, Freedman BA, Shawen SB, et al. Wound complications following the use of FiberWire in lower extremity traumatic amputations. A case series. *J Bone Joint Surg Am*. 2009;91:680-685.
5. Gardner MJ, Demetrakopoulos D, Briggs SM, Helfet DL, Lorich DG. Malreduction of the tibiofibular syndesmosis in ankle fractures. *Foot Ankle Int*. 2006;27:788-792.

SECTION VI

MISCELLANEOUS

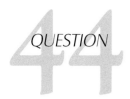
How Do You Treat Tarsal Tunnel Syndrome? What Are Your Indications for Surgical Decompression?

Christopher P. Chiodo, MD

Tarsal tunnel syndrome is an entrapment neuropathy of the posterior tibial nerve at the level of the medial ankle. Here, the nerve passes through a fibro-osseous space bordered by the tibia anteromedially and the talus and calcaneus posterolaterally. It is covered by the flexor retinaculum, also known as the laciniate ligament.

The first step in treating tarsal tunnel syndrome is to establish and confirm the diagnosis. A diagnostic triad has been described consisting of the history, physical examination, and neurodiagnostic studies. The most important component of the history is localization of symptoms—whether paresthesias, numbness, or radiation pain—in the distribution of the tibial nerve. For the physical examination, a Tinel's test may be positive with manual percussion along the tarsal tunnel. With regard to neurodiagnostic studies, the diagnostic sensitivity of sensory-nerve conduction studies ranges from 90% to 100%.[1] Mixed-nerve conduction studies have a sensitivity of 86% and superior specificity, and therefore are also helpful.[2]

In addition, I routinely obtain a magnetic resonance (MR) scan in all patients. Frey and Kerr reported abnormal findings in 85% of patients with tarsal tunnel syndrome.[3] MR can detect an underlying neoplastic process, which should always be considered in the differential diagnosis (Figure 44-1). It can also detect other diagnoses, such as varicosities, tenosynovitis, an accessory soleus muscle, and posterior tibial tendon pathology.

I usually attempt some form of nonoperative treatment. If there is any hindfoot malalignment, then appropriate orthoses are prescribed with medial or lateral hindfoot posting. While hindfoot valgus can put the posterior tibial nerve under tension, hindfoot varus may result in nerve compression. If tenosynovitis is felt to play a role, a trial of nonsteroidal anti-inflammatory medications, immobilization, and/or therapy with iontophoresis may be attempted. Lastly, a single steroid injection into the tarsal tunnel may be considered. I perform this only occasionally and with great caution, given the proximity of the nerve to vascular structures and load-bearing tendons.

Figure 44-1. Coronal MR image of lipoma extending into the tarsal tunnel.

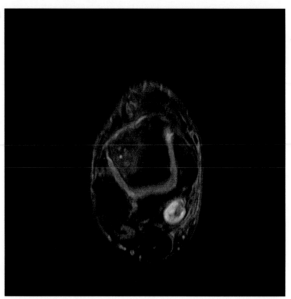

Figure 44-2. Standard extensile skin incision.

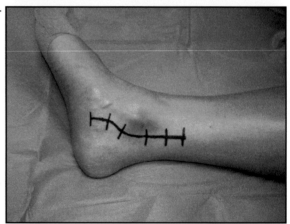

In the setting of persistent symptoms, surgical release of the tarsal tunnel is indicated. I will usually allow 6 to 12 weeks for patients to respond to nonoperative management, and many patients present having already had this. I agree with the findings of Skalley and colleagues that an adequate incision is critical to the success of the procedure.[4] These authors reported that an inadequate incision is associated with a poor outcome. As such, my incision begins approximately 8 cm medial to the medial malleolus and 1 to 2 cm posterior to the posterior border of the tibia (Figure 44-2). It extends longitudinally distally. At the tip of the medial malleolus, it curves gently anterior and then distally, such that the distal tarsal tunnel and first branch of the lateral plantar nerve ("Baxter's nerve")[5] can be released. I routinely release Baxter's nerve during a tarsal tunnel release. Bipolar electrocautery is used for hemostasis. Also, a thigh tourniquet is used.

The deep dissection is carried out under loupe magnification and begins proximally. Here, the crural fascia is identified and divided in line with the skin incision using Steven's scissors. The deep release is continued distally until the laciniate ligament, or

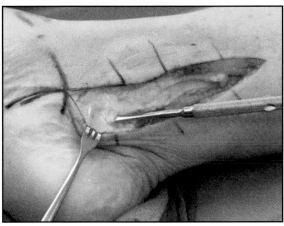

Figure 44-3. Flexor retinaculum (laciniate ligament).

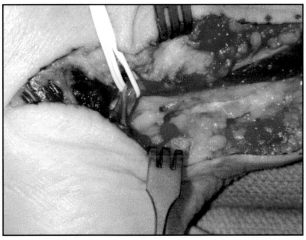

Figure 44-4. Transverse venous branches crossing the tarsal tunnel.

flexor retinaculum, is encountered. This structure is a contiguous distal thickening of the crural fascia. It is divided in line with the skin incision, taking great care to protect the underlying neurovascular structures (Figure 44-3). Again, a complete release is essential and must extend adequately distally.

Deep to the crural fascia and laciniate ligament, the nerve and accompanying vascular structures are encountered. Unless there has been previous surgery or substantial trauma, a formal neurolysis is not typically performed. Often, small venous branches are noted crossing over the tibial nerve, and these are carefully ligated and released (Figure 44-4). However, longitudinal varicosities, if present, are not resected and are treated simply by decompressing the overlying fascia.

This completes the formal component of the tarsal tunnel release. As noted, I also routinely release the first branch of the lateral plantar nerve. To accomplish this, the superficial and deep fascia of the abductor hallucis muscle are circumferentially released (Figure 44-5). The latter entails gentle mobilization of the muscle belly with a right angle retractor. Deep to the deep fascia, a fat stripe indicates the course of the nerve. The nerve does not need to be formally exposed. This avoids unnecessary manipulation of the nerve. The superior edge of the abductor fascia, where the superficial and deep components meet, is often quite rigid and can be a distinct site of compression.

Figure 44-5. Release of Baxter's nerve with exposure of the abductor hallucis muscle distally.

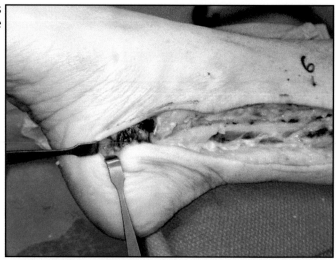

Figure 44-6. Final release extending from proximal to distal.

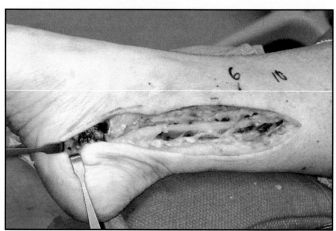

At this point, the release is examined from proximal to distal to confirm its adequacy (Figure 44-6). If there is concomitant tenosynovitis, a tenosynovectomy is performed at this point. The tourniquet is then let down and meticulous hemostasis obtained with the bipolar electrocautery unit. This is a critical step as it decreases the likelihood of scar formation and recurrent nerve compression. Further, it minimizes the chance of developing a postoperative hematoma, which can result in wound dehiscence and infection. Despite research into the importance of an appropriate preoperative skin preparation, I feel that avoiding hematoma is as important as optimizing the preoperative skin prep.

The subcutaneous tissues and skin are then closed in layers. The crural fascia and laciniate ligament are not closed. A dry sterile compression dressing is applied. I do recommend at least 2 weeks of immobilization and protected weight bearing, primarily to optimize wound healing.

References

1. Os SJ, Meyer RD. Entrapment neuropathies of the tibial nerve. *Neurol Clin.* 1993;17(3):593-615.
2. Galardi G, Amadio S, Maderna L, et al. Electrophysiologic studies in tarsal tunnel syndrome. Diagnostic reliability of motor distal latency, mixed nerve and sensory nerve conduction studies. *Am J Phys Med Rehabil.* 1994;73(3):193-198.
3. Frey C, Kerr R. Magnetic resonance imaging and the evaluation of tarsal tunnel syndrome. *Foot Ankle Int.* 1993;14(3):159-164.
4. Skalley TC, Schon LC, Hinton RY, Myerson MS. Clinical results following revision tibial nerve release. *Foot Ankle Int.* 1994;15(7):360-367.
5. Baxter DE, Pfeffer GB. Treatment of chronic heel pain by surgical release of the first branch of the lateral plantar nerve. *Clin Orthop.* 1992;279:229-236.

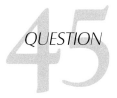

HOW DO YOU EVALUATE AND TREAT EXERTIONAL COMPARTMENT SYNDROME OF THE LEG?

Johnny Lin, MD and Samuel McArthur, MD

Exertional or chronic compartment syndrome (CCS) is primarily a disorder found in young, active adults. The etiology of CCS has not been completely elucidated. Multiple investigators have noted increased muscle and interstitial fluid volumes with activity[1] as well as elevated calf compartment pressures[1-3] in patients with CCS. Diminished perfusion and altered metabolism with improvement after fasciotomy have also been demonstrated in CCS.[1] The relative contributions of mechanical compression, decreased blood flow, and increased lactic acid production to pain and dysfunction is as yet unresolved. The most commonly involved compartments are the anterior and deep posterior, which account for 75% of cases.[4] The posterior tibial tendon has been described as residing in its own compartment, and some have referred to as many as 7 compartments[2] in the calf. However, I have not found this to be practical or necessary and routinely consider only the 4 classic compartments (anterior, lateral, superficial posterior, and deep posterior). The majority of cases are associated with recreational activities. Running and cross country skiing are prototypical; however, work-related cases have also been reported.[2]

The diagnosis of CCS can be quite challenging, with the majority of cases having a significant delay in diagnosis. Detmer et al reported an average of 22 months from onset to evaluation by an orthopedist.[2] Patient history is critical to the diagnosis, with the key feature being reproduction of symptoms following exertion. Common symptoms include dull discomfort, pain, and the sensation of fullness or pressure within an anatomical compartment following exertion. Neurologic complaints are present in approximately 17% of patients. Problems can include both weakness and paresthesia, are usually transient, and should be related to the distribution of a specific compartment and its traversing sensory and motor nerves. Baseline symptoms that are not accompanied by exacerbations with increased activity are not consistent with CCS. As the syndrome worsens, the diagnosis becomes more difficult as patients may begin reporting prolonged discomfort following exertion or exacerbation of symptoms with daily activities alone. Care must be taken to differentiate exertional worsening from that occurring with a change in position, as this finding is more consistent with neurogenic (spinal) claudication. Physical examination findings in the office can be fairly unremarkable, but in some cases, there is palpable tenderness over the affected compartment. Tenderness over the medial border of the tibia itself is concerning for stress fracture and can be differentiated on the basis of plain films or advanced imaging with either bone scan or magnetic resonance imaging (MRI). Careful evaluation of sensory and motor function of the involved compartment is necessary, but actual deficit is rare. Pulses should be intact with CCS. Patients with signs of decreased perfusion should undergo further evaluation for peripheral vascular disease as a potential cause for exertional limb pain. Common signs associated with acute compartment syndrome such as tense compartments and pain with passive stretch occur with more marked elevations in compartment pressure and are not consistent with CCS. Radiographic imaging such as plain films, MRI, computed tomography, or bone scans is typically used to rule out other potential causes of leg pain but may be normal in the diagnosis of CCS.

Definitive diagnosis of CCS can be aided with the use of compartment pressure measurements when the history and physical examination findings are equivocal and the diagnosis is still in question. I also use this modality when considering surgery to assure myself and the patient that they are a good candidate for surgical treatment. There are many acceptable devices for measuring compartment pressures. Wick and slit catheters have the advantage of being able to remain in place for multiple measurements and allow the possibility of dynamic pressure measurement. However, not all patients are able to reproduce symptoms with limited exercises such as seated dorsiflexion and plantarflexion, and it may be it difficult to maintain these catheters with more rigorous activities. Stryker needle devices (Stryker Instruments, Kalamazoo, MI) have the advantages of familiarity and availability but require a separate puncture for each measurement. I typically infiltrate the site with 2 to 3 mL of lidocaine, being careful to adequately anesthetize the skin and deep soft tissues to the level of the fascia. As long as this area is clearly marked with a surgical pen, I have not found use of the Stryker to be a problem. Two of the more frequently cited sets of objective values for diagnosing CCS are those by Rorabeck et al and Pedowitz et al.[3,4] Rorabeck noted significant overlap with normal controls, however, and I typically use those proposed by Pedowitz as a guideline (Table 45-1). I take 2 measurements—one pre-exercise and one 5 minutes after. With the patient resting supine, the device is equilibrated at the level where the measurement will be performed and then carefully inserted into the compartment. Ideally, the knee and ankle should be in the same position for both measurements. Pressures should quickly return to normal in a patient without CCS, and I see little value in the addition of dynamic or early, less than 5-minute, postexercise measurements.

The limited available data suggest that conservative treatment of CCS is unsuccessful unless patients are willing to strictly limit their activities. The goal of surgical treatment is to release the fascia of the diseased compartment. There are numerous methods for fascial release ranging from fibulectomy to "minimally invasive" vertical or transverse incisions. I believe that fibulectomy is unnecessarily morbid, and techniques using extremely limited or transverse incisions should be approached with caution as lack of visualization can lead to an inadequate release or neurovascular injury. For anterior and lateral compartment release, I prefer to use 2 5- to 6-cm longitudinal incisions over the intermuscular septa to release the anterior and lateral compartments (Figure 45-1). The superficial peroneal nerve is identified and protected in the distal incision (Figure 45-2).

<u>Table 45-1</u>

Pedowitz Criteria for Chronic Compartment Syndrome

Resting pressure	>15 mm Hg
1 minute post-exercise	≥30 mm Hg
5 minutes post-exercise	≥20 mm Hg

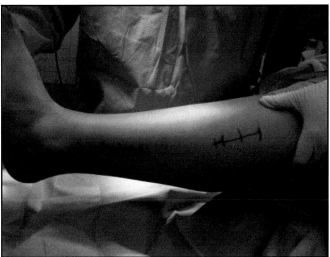

Figure 45-1. Intraoperative photograph illustrating incisions for release of the anterior and lateral compartments.

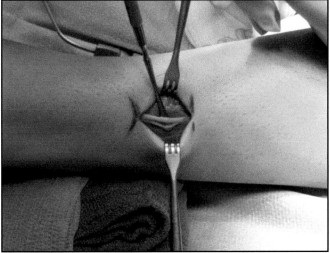

Figure 45-2. Superficial peroneal nerve is visualized and protected within the distal incision for release of the lateral compartment.

Figure 45-3. Intraoperative photograph illustrating a 3- to 4-cm incision posterior to the medial border of the tibia for release of the posterior compartment.

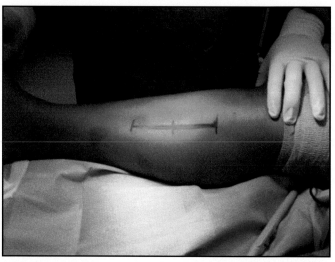

The dissection is then carried anteriorly toward the crest of the tibia and to allow release of the fascia over the anterior compartment. The lateral compartment fascia is released by dissecting posteriorly and then incising the fascia in line with the fibula. The intervening fascia between the proximal and distal incisions is released under direct visualization by elevating the subcutaneous fat and skin between the incisions and connecting the proximal and distal fascial releases. Release of the posterior compartment requires a third incision 3 to 4 cm posterior to the medial border of the tibia (Figure 45-3). The saphenous vein and nerve are identified and protected while the superficial fascia is incised. If deep release is also required, the overlying soleus is elevated, the neurovascular bundle identified, and the deep fascia over the tibialis posterior divided. Meticulous hemostasis is required to prevent hematoma and scar formation. The incision is closed in a subcuticular fashion. The patient can begin weight bearing as tolerated the day of surgery and should cease crutch use by 3 to 5 days. Elevation and compression are important for controlling swelling in the immediate postoperative period. Sports and other vigorous activities can be resumed as soon as the wounds have healed, usually 3 to 4 weeks. Consistent improvements in symptoms and activity levels have been demonstrated with similar regimens.[2,4] In several series, the results of deep posterior release have been less predictable than those for anterior or lateral compartments. I believe inadequate release is responsible for many of these failures and underscores the necessity of adequate operative exposure.

References

1. Qvarfordt P, Christenson JT, Eklöf B, Ohlin P, Saltin B. Intramuscular pressure, muscle blood flow, and skeletal muscle metabolism in chronic anterior tibial compartment syndrome. *Clin Orthop.* 1983;179:284-291.
2. Detmer DE, Sharpe K, Sufit RL, Girdley FM. Chronic compartment syndrome: diagnosis, management, and outcomes. *Am J Sports Med.* 1985;13:162-170.
3. Rorabeck CH, Bourne RB, Fowler PJ, Finlay JB, Nott L. The role of tissue pressure measurement in diagnosing chronic anterior compartment syndrome. *Am J Sports Med.* 1988;16:143-146.
4. Pedowitz RA, Hargens AR, Mubarak SJ, Gershuni DH. Modified criteria for the objective diagnosis of chronic syndrome of the leg. *Am J Sports Med.* 1990;18:35-40.

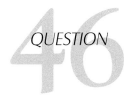

DOES COMPARTMENT SYNDROME OF THE FOOT REALLY EXIST? HOW SHOULD I TREAT IT?

Michael S. Pinzur, MD

The clinical entity of compartment syndrome in the 2 compartments of the forearm and 4 compartments of the leg is well accepted. Delay in diagnosis leads to paralysis, deformity, and appreciable permanent disability. The first question that must be addressed is whether the anatomy of the foot would support a similar pathologic process. Manoli and Weber have described 4 compartments in the foot that encase the entire muscle bellies of the intrinsic muscles of the foot with facial connective tissue.[1] The question is whether a crush injury with or without bony fracture can produce sufficient bleeding and/or swelling to create an outflow obstruction that is sufficient to impair arterial inflow, leading to muscle death and late joint contracture. The simple answer is yes. The complex answer is how do we diagnose this specific clinical entity, and is the morbidity of treatment worse than the natural history?

Compartment syndrome can develop in the foot following crush injury or closed fracture. Following some critical threshold of bleeding and/or swelling into the fixed space compartments, arterial pulse pressure is insufficient to overcome the osmotic tissue pressure gradient, leading to cell death. The complicating factor is related to the magnitude of the force of the crush injury. The amount of swelling or bleeding has to be sufficient to impair arterial inflow, while not being of sufficient magnitude to produce an open injury, which decompresses the pressure within the affected compartments. When the injury is open, we then attribute the late disability primarily to the crushing injury to the involved muscles.

To make diagnosis even more complex, we do not fully understand how frequently the crush injury and resultant swelling lead to neurogenic pain (ie, complex regional pain syndrome [CRPS] or reflex sympathetic dystrophy [RSD]). Both compartment syndrome and CRPS are frequently initiated by a crush injury with resultant swelling. How often is the pain associated with CRPS actually secondary to an overlooked compartment syndrome of the foot? How many patients with residual compartment syndrome are wrongly diagnosed with CRPS?

Figure 46-1. (A) This patient returned to clinic 10 days after sustaining a closed calcaneus fracture that was treated in a well-padded splint. (B) Two weeks later, he developed a full thickness skin loss. Was this a compartment syndrome of the foot or a simple fracture blister?

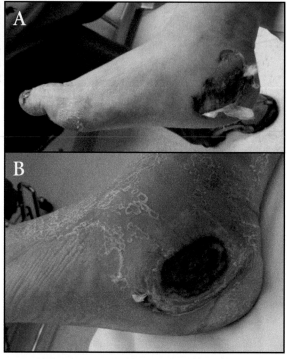

What is the natural history of untreated compartment syndrome in the foot? What is the late outcome of many patients with CRPS? The answer is that the clinical sequela of both conditions can be strikingly similar. To avoid operating on every patient with RSD, we need to consider the natural history of untreated compartment syndrome of the foot.

The acute pain associated with missed, or untreated, compartment syndrome of the foot eventually resolves to some degree. Patients typically develop joint stiffness and clawing of the toes. This sounds remarkably similar to some patients with CRPS. How can we treat these patients? Aggressive physical therapy, nerve blocks, and accommodative footwear often alleviate many of the symptoms. When the deformities of the toes are sufficiently symptomatic, we can offer reconstructive claw toe surgery, fusion of the hallux metatarsophalangeal joint, and/or excision of the scarred nonfunctional muscle.[2]

Is there a worst case scenario associated with compartment syndrome of the foot? The patient in Figure 46-1 developed significant soft tissue swelling of the heel associated with a closed calcaneus fracture that was initially treated with a well-padded splint and compression dressing. The fracture was treated with fine wire external fixation. The blister identified in Figure 46-1 progressed to a full-thickness skin loss that healed by secondary intention. Was this clinical entity a compartment syndrome associated with the closed calcaneus fracture, or was this a simple fracture blister?

What clinical outcomes can we expect with prompt correct diagnosis of compartment syndrome of the foot and urgent surgical decompression? In the best case scenario, the wounds heal with minimal scarring, intrinsic muscle function is maintained, and the patient exhibits little late difficulty with footwear. Unfortunately, this optimal favorable outcome is the exception rather than the rule. The resultant scars and necessary skin grafting can be worse than the untreated patient.

Does compartment syndrome of the foot exist? The evidence and my personal experience would suggest that the answer is yes. Can one distinguish compartment syndrome of the foot from acute neurogenic crush injury that will eventually lead to CRPS or RSD? That is a very difficult question to answer, due to the similar common endpoints of both clinical entities. For these reasons, I choose to accept the natural history method of treatment. We use compression dressings and cold therapy. If the treatment is noninterventional observation, the patient perceives his or her less-than-favorable outcome as a consequence of the injury. If one performs aggressive surgery and achieves a similar unfavorable outcome, the patient associates this poor outcome with the surgery and the surgeon.

References

1. Manoli A II, Weber TG. An anatomic study with special reference to release of the calcaneal compartment. *Foot Ankle.* 1990;10:267-275.
2. Perry MD, Manoli A II. Reconstruction of the foot after leg or foot compartment syndrome. *Foot Ank Clin.* 2006;11:191-201.

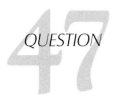

WHAT ARE SOME TECHNIQUES YOU USE IN TREATING FOOT AND ANKLE INJURIES IN YOUR PATIENTS WITH OSTEOPOROSIS?

Carroll P. Jones, MD

Osteoporosis is a systemic disease characterized by a decrease in bone mineral density (BMD) and a disruption of the bone microarchitecture. For women, it has been defined by the World Health Organization as a decrease in BMD 2.5 standard deviations below peak bone mass for the average healthy 20-year-old female. There are many causes of osteoporosis, and it affects approximately 28 million Americans. The vast majority (80%) are women. For individuals older than 65 years of age, it is a contributing factor in 75% of fractures caused by low-energy falls.[1]

The patients that I treat for osteoporotic foot and ankle fractures present many challenges. Most are elderly with multiple medical comorbidities, and many are malnourished. The condition of the soft tissues is often poor and their vascular status may be diminished. These factors all contribute to a lower healing potential. Furthermore, difficulties with balance, loss in strength, and reduced mental faculties may play a role in noncompliance with weight-bearing restrictions.

The indications for surgery are not much different than they are for patients with similar injuries with normal bone quality. Displaced unstable fracture patterns are typically treated surgically. Certainly the threshold to operate may be different for certain injuries. For example, a minimally displaced Lisfranc injury may be more appropriately treated nonoperatively in an elderly patient with poor bone quality compared to a similar injury in a young athlete.

Nonoperative treatment for osteoporotic fractures usually requires closer follow up and longer periods of immobilization. There is a decline in fracture healing capacity with the aging process. The strength of callus formation has been shown to be weaker in osteoporotic bone in experimental animal models.[2] In my experience, removable fracture boots are often cumbersome and difficult for elderly patients, and a below-knee cast may be easier to manage in some respects. However, especially for patients with tenuous soft

Figure 47-1. A 92-year-old female fell at home and sustained this comminuted osteoporotic trimalleolar ankle fracture subluxation.

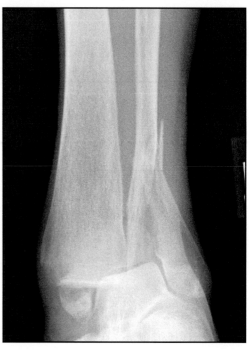

tissues, I typically change the cast every 1 to 2 weeks to allow close monitoring of the skin. Frequent radiographs in the initial treatment phase are important to ensure that acceptable alignment is maintained.

For unstable fracture patterns that require surgery, the challenging goal is achieving stable bone fixation and minimizing soft-tissue disruption. Osteoporotic fractures most often occur in soft cancellous metaphyseal bone, which has a larger area for turnover compared to denser cortical diaphyseal bone. Typically occurring in periarticular regions, this presents the additional challenge of limited bone stock available for fixation purchase.

The most common osteoporotic injuries that I see in my practice are distal tibial and ankle fractures. For these injuries, locked-plate fixation has revolutionized surgical treatment. The majority of the ankle fractures include a distal, often comminuted, lateral malleolus. Precontoured locking fibular plates are ideal for this indication (Figures 47-1 and 47-2). In addition to allowing more fixation in a smaller area compared to the traditional one-third tubular plate, there tends to be less soft-tissue irritation. The plates are lower profile and the locked screws are seated flush with the plate. I typically use 3 to 4 locking screws distally and 3 to 4 nonlocking screws proximally in the fibula for the typical Weber B fracture pattern. The soft quality of the bone often precludes the ability to apply an effective lag screw. I try to avoid disrupting the periosteum around the fracture and can often restore length and rotation with fairly minimal bony dissection.

The medial malleolus is equally challenging. The bone is often soft and comminuted with minimal bone stock for fixation. My preference is to use 2 fully-threaded "positional" cancellous screws (see Figures 47-1 and 47-2). An alternative method is a small plate contoured around the tip of the medial malleolus. However, this may be problematic if adequate low-tension soft-tissue coverage is not feasible, as is often the case in this

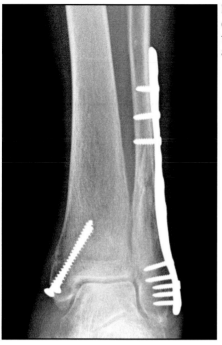

Figure 47-2. Postoperative anteroposterior radiograph demonstrating restored ankle alignment and healed fractures treated with lateral malleolar locking plate and fully threaded screws in medial malleolus.

location. A third option is the use of a tension band technique. Strong suture or wire applied through the deltoid or around bent Kirschner wires distally and secured to a screw postproximally may be effective if screw or plate fixation is deemed inadequate or impossible.

Unstable midfoot injuries are also challenging in patients with osteoporosis. Comminuted fractures at the metatarsal bases are difficult to treat with screw or pin fixation alone. I prefer to use minifragment (2.4 or 2.7 mm) locking plates applied using a "bridge" technique. For the medial column, the plate is secured proximal to the tarsometatarsal joints in the cuneiform bones (typically locked screws) and distally in the metatarsals (standard nonlocking screws). The plates can be left in place long term but may be removed no sooner than 4 months postoperatively. I typically permit weight bearing 2 months after surgery.

Postoperatively, physical therapy is initiated to facilitate mobilization, even if patients are nonweight bearing. I usually allow patients to at least put the weight of the cast on the ground for balance until the fracture is healed. Nutritional specialists are consulted in the hospital for those patients that are identified as malnourished. The majority of patients with osteoporosis will need calcium supplementation (1000 to 1500 mg/day), a multivitamin, and bisphosphonate treatment. I usually defer the medications to the patient's primary care physician.[3]

References

1. Lucas TS, Einhorn TA. Osteoporosis: the role of the orthopaedist. *J Am Acad Orthop Surg.* 1993;1:48-56.
2. Ekeland A, Engesoeter LB, Langeland N. Influence of age on mechanical properties of healing fractures and intact bones in rats. *Acta Orthop Scand.* 1982;53:527-534.
3. Cornell C. Internal fracture fixation in patients with osteoporosis. *J Am Acad Orthop Surg.* 2003;11:109-119.

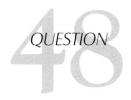

WHAT ARE SOME TECHNIQUES USED IN TREATING FOOT AND ANKLE INJURIES IN PATIENTS WITH DIABETES?

Keith L. Wapner, MD

The most critical component when evaluating a diabetic patient with a foot and ankle injury is to determine the presence and extent of any underlying neuropathy. All 3 components of diabetic neuropathy—sensory, autonomic, and motor—need to be identified and evaluated. Development of Charcot arthropathy following a diabetic injury is the most common cause of severe complications. The presence of neuropathy is generally a good indicator of the risk of developing Charcot complications. However, even without the identifiable sensory neuropathy of the skin, it is possible to have a Charcot deformity develop. It is also important to evaluate the vascular status of the patient to determine the neurovascular blood supply to undergo surgery if necessary.[1]

Physical examination should include neurologic evaluation with a Semmes-Weinstein 5.07 monofilament to determine the presence or absence of underlying sensory neuropathy. Testing should be done bilaterally. First test each of the sensory nerves—the sural laterally on the foot out to the fourth and fifth toes, the superficial peroneal on the dorsum of the foot and out to the dorsum of the second through fourth toes, the deep peroneal in the first web space, and the saphenous medially along the foot out to the dorsum of the first toe. All 3 components of the posterior tibial nerve should be tested—the calcaneal branches on the plantar surface of the heel, the medial plantar nerve below the first through third metatarsal and toes, and the lateral below the fourth and fifth metatarsal and toes.

Assessment of the blood supply to the foot and ankle starts with the palpation of the posterior tibial artery at the level of the tarsal tunnel and the dorsalis pedis pulse at the dorsum of the midfoot. Approximately 15% of people with normal circulation do not have a dorsalis pedis. Another guide to adequate blood flow is to assess if there is still hair growth on the dorsum of the toes. If the pedal pulses are not palpable, then an ischemic index Doppler evaluation should be performed. Often this is not feasible with an acute injury, but this should be obtained if there has been recent evaluation of the pedal pulses. When ordering the ischemic index, you must specify not only for an arterial brachial index (ABI), but also request that the dorsalis pedis be tested and toe waves be tested. An ABI of greater than 0.5 is a good indicator of adequate flow for surgical healing when paired with a total albumin of greater than 3.0 and a total lymphocyte count of greater than 1500.[2,3]

Ligamentous injuries can be as devastating as bony injuries because they can also lead to the development of Charcot arthropathy. In a diabetic who presents with a history of injury, a normal x-ray and minimal pain does not necessarily preclude a significant injury. You must remember that because of the neuropathy, the patient may be able to tolerate the exam and weight bear without difficulty. You can never safely rely on the patient's complaints of minimal pain as an indicator of the severity of injury.

In evaluating an acute injury, if there is the presence of swelling or ecchymosis, the best course of action is to treat this aggressively with complete immobilization (Figure 48-1A). Soft tissue injuries such as Lisfranc sprains and ankle sprains will often progress to dislocations because of the lack of sensory feedback. A patient with neuropathy does not get the normal pain feedback that would cause them to limit the stress on the injured extremity. They will continue to walk and the further cyclical loading of the foot or ankle will lead to further disruption of the injured ligamentous structures. This will ultimately lead to complete disruption of the ligaments and surrounding joint capsule and a complete dislocation of the joint may occur.

Once the dislocation occurs, the patient may still have no pain but will present with a grossly swollen, red, warm extremity. This may be accompanied with secondary bony destruction on radiographs and be misdiagnosed as an infection. These patients are often admitted to the hospital and started on intravenous antibiotics but allowed to continue weight bearing (Figures 48-1B and 48-1C). When the clinical picture does not improve, an orthopedic consult is ordered for a bone biopsy. At that time, a careful history can disclose the timeline that points to this being a Charcot joint rather than an infection. Oftentimes, 24 to 48 hours of strict nonweight bearing will lead to a decrease in swelling and erythema and help convince the medical service that a biopsy is not required.

This cascade of events can usually be avoided by aggressively treating these patients with total contact casting at the onset of injury.

In the treatment of fractures, a stable reduction is required (Figure 48-1D). Again, the postoperative immobilization is critical as these patients do not experience normal pain. Careful patient instructions to exercise the need for nonweight bearing must be emphasized (Figures 48-1E and 48-1F). If the fracture is acute and the patient's vascular status is satisfactory, immediate surgery can be performed. If the fracture or dislocation is already showing signs of a Charcot reaction with significant erythema, swelling, and bony destruction, a period of total contact casting to settle down the Charcot reaction preoperatively will increase the likelihood of a successful surgical outcome. We refer to the Eichenholtz classification of Charcot progression. Stage 1 is fragmentation and we try to avoid surgery at this stage. Stage 2 is coalescence and surgery can be considered at this stage and will have a better chance of success without worsening the fragmentation. Stage 3 is consolidation and is the safest time for elective surgery.[3]

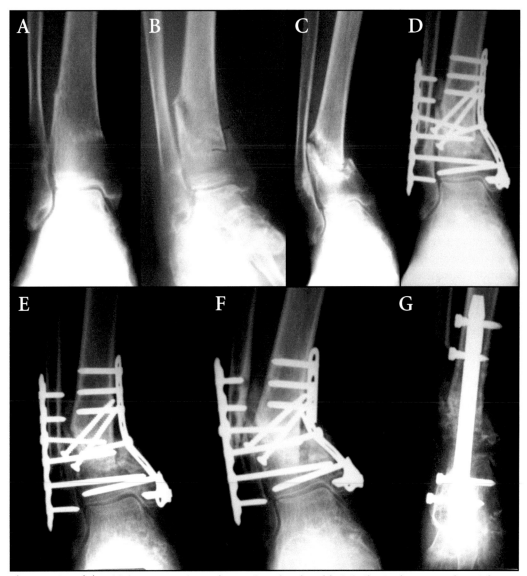

Figure 48-1. (A) Initial presentation after a "sprained ankle." Patient given an aircast brace. (B) Patient returned to emergency room 2 weeks later with increased swelling but no pain. Switched to a fracture walking boot. (C) Patient presents to his orthopedist 6 weeks postinjury because of increased swelling, heat, and deformity but no pain. Patient advised to have immediate surgery. (D) Initial postoperative x-rays. Patient placed in a cast and advised to be nonweight bearing. (E) Patient returns 4 weeks postoperatively. Claims he was not weight bearing but the bottom of the cast is broken down. Patient is recasted and again instructed to be nonweight bearing. (F) Patient returns at 8 weeks because the cast got wet and he removed it a week ago and now the leg "looks different" but doesn't hurt, so he thought he could just wait for his appointment. (G) Patient referred to Foot and Ankle Specialist and salvaged with an intramedullary rod. Initial treatment of the injury with a total contact cast, nonweight bearing with a roll-about device may have prevented this cascade of injury.

The general rule in our practice is that we double the period of immobilization in a patient with diabetic neuropathy. We also emphasize the use of the devices such as a roll-about to help assist these patients in remaining nonweight bearing (Figure 48-1G). Because of the lack of sensory feedback, the patient will often present stating that he or she has not walked on the cast but the bottom of the cast is broken down because he or she has not felt the pressure. By using a device such as a roll-about, it allows them to kneel on the extremity rather than push off on the extremity.

The most important component of management of diabetic injuries is a high index of suspicion. Aggressive cast immobilization despite normal x-ray findings, the use of total contact casting to prevent secondary skin injury or ulceration, and weekly cast changes in the initial weeks after injury will increase your chances of successful management. Careful vascular and nutritional assessment is essential in patients that need to undergo surgery. In the presence of active Charcot reaction, preoperative total contact casting until coalescence begins will increase the odds of success. Frequent cast changes in the initial weeks of treatment and prolonged immobilization will assist in preventing the development of Charcot arthropathy.

References

1. Pinzur MS. Current concepts review: Charcot arthropathy of the foot and ankle. *Foot Ankle Int.* 2007;28(8):952-959.
2. Pinzur MS. Amputation level selection in the diabetic foot. *Clin Orthop Relat Res.* 1993;(296):68-70.
3. Robinson AH, Pasapula C, Brodsky JW. Surgical aspects of the diabetic foot. *J Bone Joint Surg Br.* 2009;91(1): 1-7.

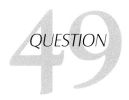

Do I Need to Use Bone Graft for Foot or Ankle Surgery? Which Graft Should I Use—Autologous or Allograft?

Christopher Bibbo, DO, FACS, FAAOS

The foot and ankle surgeon commonly encounters situations where patients possess risk factors for bony healing problems (Table 49-1), have had same-site failed surgeries, or have bone defects that will require restoration of bone stock.[1-3]

To begin, common sense is paramount in treating patients and assessing risk factors. When it appears that bone will be needed, currently there is no equal substitute. The decision whether allograft or autograft is needed is based on patient stratification, surgical needs, and clinical situation (Figure 49-1). It is the author's preference that when bone graft is needed, autograft is the bone source of choice. Allograft is certainly an acceptable bone graft in patients where structural material is needed to restore length, fill defects, or correct deformity in an area that is richly vascularized (such as cancellous bone or cortical bone with a large muscle bed over it) in patients who are not at risk for bone healing problems. For example, in a normal, healthy young patient in whom an Evans procedure or other similar lateral column lengthening is being performed, allograft is certainly acceptable. If the patient has a high risk for a nonunion, then autograft is preferred. In patients where the area is not richly vascularized, not only do we need bone, but we need osteoprogenitor cells; both osteoinductive and osteoconductive properties are needed in the bone graft. In this instance, autograft is again the preference (Figure 49-2). Whether it is richly vascularized or not richly vascularized, in an anatomical area where there is a defect or deformity in a patient that has significant risk factors for bone healing problems, autograft is preferred. The use of bone substitutes in place of bone is unacceptable (eg, photo-oxidized bovine bone or polyglycolic/polylactate materials are unsuitable in place of human bone).[4,5]

A common question arises in patients who are in the ambulatory setting, have low risk factors, and are undergoing procedures that have known risk for nonunions (eg, talar navicular fusions, metatarsophalangeal joint fusion, and Lapidus procedures).

Table 49-1

List of Risk Factors for Poor Bone Healing for Which Bone Grafting May Be Indicated. The Choice of Graft Is Influenced by Surgical Indication and Technique

• Smoking	• Immunosuppression
• Diabetes	• Chronic infections
• High-energy injury	• Suboptimal inflow
• Multiple surgeries	• Collagen disorders
• History of delayed/nonunion	• Multiple medical comorbidities
• Alcohol abuse	• Disorders of calcium homeostasis

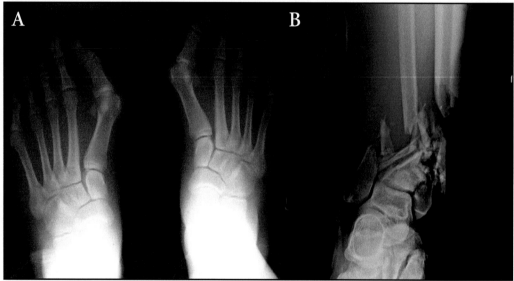

Figure 49-1. Two starkly contrasting cases. (A) Elective first tarsometatarsal fusion in a healthy young adult where bone graft is not needed, compared to (B) a high-energy open pilon fracture in a smoker that will require bone grafting and osteobiologic augmentation.

It is a common question to ask if there is anything to be done to specifically enhance the union rates in these situations and if bone is actually required. My answer to this question is that proper surgical technique can generally suffice without the use of additional bone. Additional bone that can be harvested locally can be used if there is a defect. If a question still arises, we use adjuvant modalities such as platelet-rich plasma in my practice.[6] The assessment of the need for bone graft, as well as adjuvant osteobiologic agents, has been proposed by me in my Host-Surgical Site classification system,[6] which uses a 4-category system that stratifies patients into risk classes that correlate with surgical needs for bone graft and osteobiologic adjuvants (Figures 49-3 and 49-4).

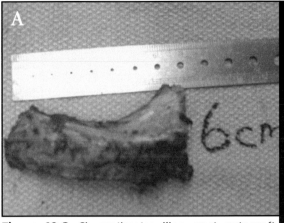
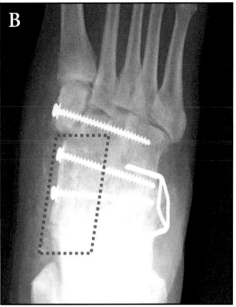

Figure 49-2. Six-centimeter iliac crest autograft used to reconstruct multiple nonunions of the medial column (outlined) in a high-risk patient. The construct fused uneventfully and the patient experienced only minimal, transient donor site morbidity.

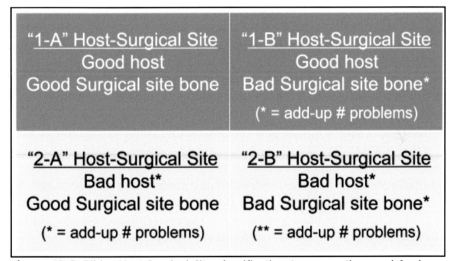

Figure 49-3. Bibbo Host-Surgical Site classification to assess the need for bone graft and osteo-adjuvants. (Reprinted with permission from Bibbo C, Hatfield PS. Platelet-rich plasma concentrate to augment bone fusion. *Foot Ankle Clin.* 2010;15(4):641-649.)

When dealing with larger reconstructions, the iliac crest remains the single best source for autologous bone graft (see Figure 49-1). Unfortunately, both clinicians and patients commonly have an aversion to harvesting iliac crest bone, with a common citation of high donor site morbidity. It is the author's experience that patients experience transient donor site discomfort, but residual sequelae and complications are very low, even in obese and morbidly obese patients (Bibbo C, unpublished data). This author's observation echoes the finding of DeOrio and Farber that the morbidity in harvesting iliac crest is actually quite low and that, when complications occur, they are transient and minor in nature[7]

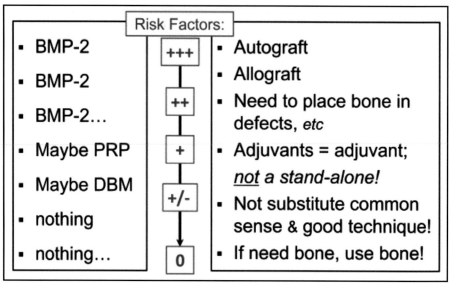

Figure 49-4. Schematic hierarchy of risk factors, bone graft, and osteobiologic adjuvants. (Reprinted with permission of Dr. C. Bibbo.)

and iliac crest bone graft should be sought when needed. Even allograft sources carry risks, particularly delayed and nonunions, infection, and fatigue fracture.[8,9] In an effort to avert the perceived morbidities from iliac crest harvest site morbidity and to avoid the use of allograft, local (more easily accessed) bone graft harvesting techniques have become popular. Sources for local bone include the calcaneus, the cuboid, medial malleolus, distal tibia, and proximal tibia. However, even "local" bone graft harvests have demonstrated a 9% complication rate.[10] The surgeon must be warned that the quality of bone from these sites is highly variable, the quantity limited, and, for the majority of foot and ankle cases, adequate. For example, in an elderly patient, the author has noted that the proximal tibia quite often yields only fatty marrow and is a poor source for bone graft. Recently, the author's observations have been confirmed histologically by other investigators who demonstrated that proximal tibial graft sites yield a more fatty marrow than the iliac crest, which consistently yields a graft with a robust level of cellular activity.[11]

The most richly vascularized and highly populated area (with stem cells) is still the iliac crest. As the body grows older, the areas for reserves of stem cells decreases throughout the body.[12,13] It appears that the iliac crest may be the best site for osteoprogenerative cells, but even this diminishes as aging ensues. These data do not, however, fully address the questions of precursor cell recruitment (graft cytokine levels) in the overall function of bone grafting. A "2-stage" hypothesis theory has been proposed to explain the fate of mesenchymal cells in-vitro, implicating that microenvironmental cues (soluble factors) are part of the complex biology of cellular (osteoprogenitor) differentiation and its role in bone healing.[14] Despite these data, many clinicians still use proximal tibial bone graft, despite the evidence that the iliac crest provides the most active, robust source for autologous bone. This author follows simple, sound clinical reasoning that expounds the philosophy that, in general, when bone graft is needed, the source is dictated based upon risk factors, the age of the patient, and specific needs (amount structural versus nonstructural).

All osteo-adjuvant modalities, including platelet-rich plasma, demineralized bone matrix, and bone morphogenetic protein are adjuncts to bone healing, and are not substitutes for human bone (both autograft and allograft). A simple way to stratify the assessment of patients for the need for both bone grafting and adjuvant osteobiologic agents has been proposed by me in my classification system,[6] which uses a surgical site and surgical candidate scale to assess the risk and need for adjuvant material. Adjuvants that can be used include platelet-rich plasma, demineralized bone matrix, bone morphogenetic protein, etc. The use of tricalcium sulfate materials and bone void fillers are simply bone void fillers that allow creeping substitution. Thus, they must be used in a well-contained defect in an area that is richly vascularized. Bone graft filler materials have no application in the reconstruction of cortical defects.

Conclusion

The use of bone graft in foot and ankle surgery is based on a sound, common sense assessment of the clinical situation, as well as host risk and surgical site risk factors. The traditional teaching for the use of bone graft still holds. When bone graft is needed to fill defects, span bone voids, correct alignment, and, when coupled with increasing risk factors, autogenous bone graft is to be used. The consideration that there is unacceptably high second surgery site morbidity has really not been completely substantiated, and, in the author's clinical experience, even large bone grafts in the morbidly obese patient can still result in good long-term results with minimal second site morbidity. Thus, for most purposes, in at-risk patients, autologous bone graft trumps allograft. However, there are certain situations where allograft will remain a valuable component in the surgeon's armamentarium. Risks of using allograft (frozen and freeze dried) increase depending on the size of the graft used. In large allograft constructs, incorporation of the allograft may take many months, if not years. In large foot and ankle reconstructions, allograft may be subject to fatigue failure and may also act as a nidus for inflammation and infection. At times, combinations of allograft and autograft must be used because there are limitations on the amount of autograft that can be harvested. Nonetheless, the use of any bone graft must be weighed against host risk factors (ex, smoking, diabetes), surgical site risk factors, (ex, vascularity of the area), and the demands of the proposed surgical construct. Thus, bone graft is not needed in every foot and ankle surgery, but rather it is dictated by host factors, surgical indications, as well as the surgical technique required to meet the operative demand of each individual patient.

References

1. Bibbo C, Patel DV, Haskell MD. Recombinant bone morphogenetic protein-2 (rhBMP-2) in high-risk ankle and hindfoot fusions. *Foot Ankle Int*. 2009;30:597-603.
2. Bibbo C, Bono CM, Lin SS. Union rates using autologous platelet concentrate alone and with bone graft in high-risk foot and ankle surgery patients. *J Surg Orthop Adv*. 2005;14:17-22.
3. Bibbo C, Anderson RB, Davis WH. Complications of midfoot and hindfoot arthrodesis. *Clin Orthop Relat Res*. 2001;391:45-58.
4. Adams MR, Gehrmann RM, Bibbo C, Garcia JP, Najarian RG, Patel DV. In vivo assessment of incorporation of bone graft substitute plugs in osteoarticular autograft transplant surgery. Paper presented at: American Orthopaedic Society for Sports Medicine Annual Meeting Final Program; July 15-18, 2010; Providence, RI.

5. Lin JS, Andersen LB, Juliano PJ. Effectiveness of composite bone graft substitute plugs in the treatment of chondral and osteochondral lesions of the talus. *J Foot Ankle Surg.* 2010;49(3):224-232.

6. Bibbo C, Hatfield PS. Platelet-rich plasma concentrate to augment bone fusion. *Foot Ankle Clin.* 2010;15(4):641-649.

7. DeOrio JK, Farber DC. Morbidity associated with anterior iliac crest bone grafting in foot and ankle surgery. *Foot Ankle Int.* 2005;26:147-151.

8. Mahan KT, Hillstrom HJ. Bone grafting in foot and ankle surgery. *J Am Pod Med Assoc.* 1998;88:108-118.

9. Stevenson S. Biology of bone grafts. *Orth Clin N Am.* 1999;30:543-552.

10. Raikin SM, Brislin K. Local bone graft harvested from the distal tibia or calcaneus for surgery of the foot and ankle. *Foot Ankle Int.* 2005;26:449-453.

11. Chiodo CP, Hahne J, Wilson MG, Glowacki J. Histologic differences in iliac and tibial bone graft. *Foot Ankle Int.* 2010;31:418-422.

12. Muschler GF, Nitto H, Boehm CA, Easly KA. Age- and gender-related changes in the cellularity of human bone marrow and the prevalence of osteoblastic progenitors. *J Orthop Res.* 2001;19:117-125.

13. Zhang W, Ou G, Hamrick M, et al. Age-related changes in the osteogenic differentiation potential of mouse bone marrow stromal cells. *J Bone Miner Res.* 2008;23:118-128.

14. Gregory CA, Ylostalo J, Prockop DJ. Adult bone marrow stem/progenitor cells (MSCs) are preconditioned by microenvironmental "niches" in culture: a two-stage hypothesis for regulation of MSC fate. *Sci STKE.* 2005;(294):pe37.

FINANCIAL DISCLOSURES

Dr. Jeremy A. Alland has no financial or proprietary interest in the materials presented herein.

Dr. John G. Anderson is a consultant for Bespa. He also receives research support from MMI, BioMimetic, and DePuy.

Dr. Robert B. Anderson is a consultant for and receives royalites from Wright Medical and Arthrex.

Dr. Judith Baumhauer is a paid consultant for DJ Orthopaedics, Carticept Medical, Extremity Medical, and BioMimetic Therapeutics. She also receives research support from DJ Orthopaedics.

Dr. Wayne Berberian is a consultant for RTI Biologics and he received an educational grant from Synthes.

Dr. Gregory C. Berlet is a consultant for Wright Medical Technology.

Dr. Christopher Bibbo has no financial or proprietary interest in the materials presented herein.

Dr. Donald R. Bohay is a consultant for Stryker, Biometric, MMI, and Bespa. He also receives royalties from MMI.

Dr. Eric Breitbart has no financial or proprietary interest in the materials presented herein.

Dr. Yong Chae has no financial or proprietary interest in the materials presented herein.

Dr. Christopher P. Chiodo has no financial or proprietary interest in the materials presented herein.

Dr. Jennifer Chu has no financial or proprietary interest in the materials presented herein.

Dr. Cara A. Cipriano has no financial or proprietary interest in the materials presented herein.

Dr. Bruce Cohen is a consultant for and receives royalities from Wright Medical Technology.

Dr. W. Hodges Davis received salary, royalty, or honoraria from DJO, Arthrex, Wright Medical, and Smith & Nephew. He also does supported/contracted research for Orthofix, DJO, and Wright Medical.

Dr. Nickolas G. Garbis has no financial or proprietary interest in the materials presented herein.

Dr. Jaymes D. Granata has no financial or proprietary interest in the materials presented herein.

Dr. Robert R. L. Gray has no financial or proprietary interest in the materials presented herein.

Dr. George B. Holmes, Jr is a consultant for, on the speaker's bureau for, and receives royalties from Arthrex, Inc. He is also on the editorial board for *Foot and Ankle International Journal* of the American Academy of Orthopaedic Surgeons.

Dr. Carroll P. Jones is a paid consultant for Wright Medical Technologies.

Dr. Armen S. Kelikian has no financial or proprietary interest in the materials presented herein.

Dr. Alex J. Kline has no financial or proprietary interest in the materials presented herein.

Dr. Pradeep Kodali has no financial or proprietary interest in the materials presented herein.

Dr. Steven A. Kodros has no financial or proprietary interest in the materials presented herein.

Dr. Simon Lee has no financial or proprietary interest in the materials presented herein.

Dr. Johnny Lin has no financial or proprietary interest in the materials presented herein.

Dr. Sheldon Lin is on the scientific advisory board for BMTI and is a consultant for Zimmer.

Dr. Sameer J. Lodha has no financial or proprietary interest in the materials presented herein.

Dr. Robert S. Marsh has no financial or proprietary interest in the materials presented herein.

Dr. Samuel McArthur has no financial or proprietary interest in the materials presented herein.

Dr. Scott Nemec has no financial or proprietary interest in the materials presented herein.

Dr. Shane J. Nho a consultant and receives research support from Stryker and Pivot Medical.

Dr. Daniel L. Ocel has no financial or proprietary interest in the materials presented herein.

Dr. Terrence M. Philbin has no financial or proprietary interest in the materials presented herein.

Dr. Michael S. Pinzur is a consultant for BioMimetics, Small Bone Innovations, and Wright Medical. He is also a lecturer for Smith & Nephew and Tornier.

Dr. David R. Richardson has no financial or proprietary interest in the materials presented herein.

Dr. Nicholas R. Seibert has no financial or proprietary interest in the materials presented herein.

Dr. Brian C. Toolan has no financial or proprietary interest in the materials presented herein.

Dr. Walter W. Virkus is a consultant for Stryker and Smith & Nephew.

Dr. Anand Vora is a consultant for Arthrex.

Dr. Keith L. Wapner is a consultant for Wright Medical, Small Bone Innovations, and MemoMetal Inc. He receives fellowship support to his institution from Hangar Corporation. He is also on the board for the American Orthopedic Foot and Ankle Society and the managerial board for *Foot and Ankle International*.

INDEX

Printed in the United States
by Baker & Taylor Publisher Services